The Arthritis Foundation's

Guide to Good Living With Rheumatoid Arthritis

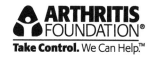

ARTHRITIS FOUNDATION®
Take Control. We Can Help.™

Published by

Arthritis Foundation

1330 West Peachtree Street

Atlanta, GA 30309

Printed in the United States of America

1st Printing 2000

Library of Congress Card Catalog Number: 00-104037

ISBN: 0-912423-21-8

Acknowledgments

The Arthritis Foundation's Guide to Good Living With Rheumatoid Arthritis is written for people who have rheumatoid arthritis, as well as for their friends, family and loved ones. Bringing this book to completion was a team effort, including the significant contributions of dedicated physicians, health-care professionals, Arthritis Foundation volunteers, writers, editors, designers and Arthritis Foundation staff.

Special acknowledgments should go to the medical editor of the book, Theodore Pincus, MD, Professor of Medicine at Vanderbilt University School of Medicine, as well as to his co-editor, Cynthia M. Kahn. The chief medical reviewer of the book is John H. Klippel, MD, Medical Director of the Arthritis Foundation. The panel of reviewers of this book are rheumatologists Joan Bathon, MD, Associate Professor of Medicine at Johns Hopkins Bayview Medical Center, Division of Rheumatology, in Baltimore, MD; Marcy Bolster, MD, Assistant Professor of Medicine, Division of Rheumatology and Immunology, at Medical University of South Carolina in Charleston, SC; and Jennifer Lewis, an Arthritis Foundation volunteer who also has rheumatoid arthritis. Additional thanks go to Gretchen Henkel, who served as a writer on the early stages of the book's development.

Editorial directors of this book are Elizabeth Axtell and Susan Bernstein. Art director and cover designer is Matthew Lennert. Interior layout design is by Jill Dible.

Table of Contents

Foreword

It is difficult, impossible really, to make comparisons among the 100 or more different forms of arthritis. Each touches the lives of persons affected in very personal and often profound ways.

By whatever standard one might choose, however, rheumatoid arthritis ranks high on the list of the most serious forms of arthritis. Although it can begin at any age – including childhood – young women in the prime of their lives are most commonly affected. Joint pain and limitations become a daily experience, and interfere with essentially all activities – those needed to simply make it through the day as well as pleasurable activities. Moreover, for most people, the arthritis becomes chronic and persists for their entire lifetime. Over the course of years, rheumatoid arthritis leads to damage to joints and deformities of hands, wrists and other joints, further limiting a person's ability to use their joints.

For many people with rheumatoid arthritis, the uncertainty of knowing what the future holds and the frustration that drugs or other approaches to treatment have provided little relief of symptoms pose major challenges. Fortunately, this situation is changing rapidly, particularly over the past decade, which has witnessed remarkable progress in the scientific understanding of rheumatoid arthritis. Research is beginning to provide important clues that have already resulted in newer, more highly effective drugs to treat the disease. Ongoing and future research will teach us a great deal about the disease, yet to be able to truly cure or even prevent rheumatoid arthritis seems a real and distinct possibility.

The Arthritis Foundation believes that the actions people with rheumatoid arthritis choose to take play a large and important role in determining the outcome of the disease, and the extent to which it impacts their lives. Education, self-help and taking personal responsibility are tools of empowerment – all keys to working effectively with physicians to achieve control of rheumatoid arthritis. This book, *The Arthritis Foundation's Guide to Good Living With Rheumatoid Arthritis,* is a resource guide for people with rheumatoid arthritis, as well as their families and loved ones, to help in the understanding of this disease, and improve their lives.

John H. Klippel, MD
Medical Director
Arthritis Foundation, Atlanta, GA

Part One

Rheumatoid Arthritis:
Understanding the Disease

Chapter 1

Understanding Arthritis:

Eradicating Myths and Exploring Treatment Models

The goal of this book is to give you strategies and information that can help you learn to live well with rheumatoid arthritis. Before we get started, though, it's necessary to take a step back and look at the big picture. This chapter may be used as a building block for understanding the complex condition known as rheumatoid arthritis.

"Arthritis" is a term derived from the Greek words "arth" (meaning joint) and "itis" (meaning inflammation). The literal meaning of the word is "joint inflammation." However, the word arthritis is often used to refer to any of the more than 100 different conditions that cause pain in the joints and tissues surrounding them, such as muscles and tendons (which connect muscles to bone). These conditions may be called forms of arthritis, musculoskeletal conditions or rheumatic diseases. In many sources – including this book – these terms are used interchangeably.

Arthritis Myths

Arthritis has been recognized for perhaps thousands of years. Unfortunately, many misconceptions about this chronic condition have been around for almost as long. We will try to debunk some of these myths about arthritis and provide some key definitions along the way.

MYTH #1: ARTHRITIS IS JUST ACHES AND PAINS

One common myth is that arthritis is just another name for the aches and pains people get as they grow older. While it is true that arthritis becomes more common as people age, arthritis may begin at any age, including childhood. Conversely, some elderly people never develop arthritis. Many forms of arthritis or musculoskeletal conditions are self-limited and get better without specific treatment. Others, such as rheumatoid arthritis, may be quite serious and may affect the body's internal organs as well as the joints.

A simple way to organize arthritis-related conditions is to group them into categories based on whether they affect only one joint

Some Arthritis Myths

Arthritis is just another name for minor aches and pains associated with aging.

Arthritis isn't really a serious health problem.

Not much can be done to help people with arthritis.

or area of the body (localized conditions) or many joints and organs over the entire body (generalized conditions), as shown in the box on page 3. Localized conditions include two subgroups. The first subgroup includes conditions that affect the soft tissues surrounding joints and bones, but do not affect the structure of joints or bones directly. These are known as soft-tissue, localized conditions, and include *tendinitis* and *bursitis*. The second subgroup includes conditions that affect one or a few joints, such as a single knee or hip. A common example of this second subgroup is osteoarthritis of a single joint, although osteoarthritis often affects more than one joint.

Likewise, generalized conditions can be divided into two subgroups. In the first subgroup, widespread muscle and soft tissue discomfort in which there is no evidence of swelling or inflammation includes a very common condition called *fibromyalgia*. Conditions in this subgroup are not associated with damage to the structure of the joints. The second subgroup includes conditions in which inflammation affects the entire body, such as rheumatoid arthritis. Other conditions in this subgroup include

gout, ankylosing spondylitis and *psoriatic arthritis*, generalized conditions of inflammation throughout the body in which joint pain is the major symptom. Other generalized inflammatory conditions include *polymyositis*, which affects primarily muscles; *systemic lupus erythematosus* (lupus), which may affect the skin, kidneys or other organs; and *vasculitis*, which may affect any organ.

These four groups of musculoskeletal conditions are not mutually exclusive, and a person may have more than one type of rheumatic disease. For example, people with rheumatoid arthritis may experience tendinitis, bursitis and fibromyalgia more commonly than people in the general population. In addition, when joints become badly damaged as a result of the chronic inflammation of rheumatoid arthritis, they are called "end stage." At this point, they may look similar to joints that have reached "end stage" in people with osteoarthritis, even though the destruction was caused by different mechanisms.

MYTH #2: ARTHRITIS ISN'T REALLY A SERIOUS HEALTH PROBLEM

Taken collectively, the various types of arthritis and rheumatic diseases are the most common chronic health condition in the population, affecting about one in every six Americans. These conditions become even more common among older people. Even in people under age 65, arthritis is a major cause of work disability. For example, fewer than 50 percent of rheumatoid arthritis patients younger than 65 who are working at the onset of the disease are still working 10 years later.

In addition, the impact of arthritis on society is substantial. By some estimates, the costs associated with arthritis may amount to $65 billion annually – putting the economic impact of arthritis on a par with a moderate recession. The costs of arthritis may be categorized into three groups: direct, indirect and intangible. *Direct* medical costs, such as physician (and other health professional) fees, charges for laboratory tests and

X-rays, drugs, assistive devices, surgeries and other costs, are the most obvious. However, a substantial part of the economic burden comes from *indirect* costs, such as lost wages due to work disability. In addition, people experience *intangible* costs, such as the need for a spouse or relative to take time off from work to bring a patient to a caregiver, travel for medical care, or money spent to remodel the home to meet the needs of a person with arthritis, and many others.

MYTH #3: NOT MUCH CAN BE DONE TO ALLEVIATE THE PAIN AND DISABILITY OF ARTHRITIS

Unfortunately, there are no cures for most chronic rheumatic conditions. You may think that little can be done to help your arthritis, but this is not true. Some improvement in the pain and loss of function is possible in almost everyone with arthritis. Furthermore, the disease process that may lead to joint destruction can be controlled effectively in most people – particularly those with rheumatoid arthritis. More can be done today to ease the pain of arthritis and to slow joint destruction than ever before.

Many people with serious types of arthritis, which were severely disabling as recently as a generation ago, are now leading full and productive lives, thanks in part to many developments, including new drugs and treatments, exercise programs, surgeries and self-management. As a person with arthritis, your future is full of possibilities that were only a dream 25 years ago.

Arthritis-Related Conditions

Localized conditions
(affect one joint or one area of the body)

- Soft tissue localized conditions (bursitis or tendinitis, for example)
- Conditions that affect one or a few joints (such as osteoarthritis)

Generalized conditions
(affect many joints or areas of the body)

- Widespread muscle/soft tissue conditions without inflammation (such as fibromyalgia)
- Inflammatory conditions usually involving joints (rheumatoid arthritis, psoriatic arthritis, gout, vasculitis and ankylosing spondylitis)

One of the most exciting changes in recent years has been the growing understanding that the patient has an important role to play in the management of his or her arthritis. This change in emphasis is sometimes referred to as a *biopsychosocial model* of disease management, to distinguish it from the traditional *biomedical model*, in which the outcomes of diseases are thought to be determined almost exclusively by the actions of health professionals. The wonderful advances in drugs, surgeries and other medical treatments are an important component of a biopsychosocial model of disease management, but this model also incorporates the key contribution of patients, families and support networks to the outcome. In the second part of this chapter, we will focus on this model, which lays the groundwork for many of the ideas expressed throughout the remainder of this book.

The Biopsychosocial Model for Arthritis Care

The biomedical model of medical care evolved in the late 19th and early 20th century and was based on the idea of identifying a single cause and cure for each disease. This model was extremely successful and is still used. It works well when doctors care for people with acute infections, such as pneumonia; acute surgical conditions, such as appendicitis; and conditions affecting a single organ, such as a heart attack. Many of our ideas and expectations of medical care are based on the success of this approach, which relies heavily on high technology tests and state-of-the-art treatments that lead to cures.

As chronic diseases and health problems have come to the forefront at the beginning of the 21st century, certain limitations of the biomedical model have become clear. First, the causes and treatments of chronic diseases are complex – there is rarely one cause or one cure. Second, people who have chronic diseases have important contributions to make to the outcomes of their disease – the results appear to be influenced as much by the actions of the patient as by the actions of the doctor or other health professionals. In fact, there is growing evidence that much of the key information for making a diagnosis, predicting the outcome and monitoring chronic disease comes directly from the patient in the form of patient histories and questionnaires. These are supplemented by the knowledge of health professionals and information gained through high technology tests.

In recognition of the importance of the patient's role, new management strategies have evolved to supplement the traditional biomedical approach. This biopsychosocial model includes the idea that chronic conditions involve an intermingling of many factors – including biological, psychological and socioeconomic – that can affect the course and outcome of disease.

This approach emphasizes that people who have chronic diseases should become knowledgeable about the consequences of disease and effects of therapy, and should understand the importance of *self-management* in disease outcomes. Self-management refers to actions by the patient that may favorably affect the course and outcome of chronic disease. By combining active self-management strategies with the information and treatment available from doctors and other health professionals, people with arthritis may experience greater benefits – such as increased pain relief and a better quality of life – than those who do not become involved in their own care. Some specific principles of the biopsychosocial approach are summarized in the accompanying box and are discussed here. These principles create the foundation on which this book is based, and they will be referred to frequently in the following chapters.

Principles of Arthritis Management

1. Each person is an individual and should be viewed as a person with a type of arthritis, rather than as a type of arthritis seen in a person.

2. There is no best treatment for everyone who has a particular type of arthritis, as each individual may respond differently to different treatments.

3. No single type of arthritis is always better or worse than another type.

4. Information and input from a person with arthritis can be as valuable in diagnosis and management as information from laboratory tests and X-rays.

5. In arthritis management, the emphasis is on improving function of joints and relieving pain.

6. Your doctor and health-care team need your involvement to help you to the fullest extent. People with arthritis and health professionals are partners in care.

7. Something can always be done to improve the situation for a person with arthritis.

I. EACH PERSON IS AN INDIVIDUAL AND MUST BE VIEWED AS A PERSON WITH A TYPE OF ARTHRITIS, RATHER THAN AS A TYPE OF ARTHRITIS IN A PERSON.

When a doctor deals with an acute problem, such as a specific type of pneumonia, there is usually a standard course of treatment that varies little from person to person. While each patient's case is unique, in acute events, the biomedical model usually works well. However, in a chronic process such as arthritis, a more individualized approach is needed. Each person may need a different combination of medications, exercise, therapy and devices to achieve the best quality of life. There is no single approach to any type of chronic arthritis that is invariably better than another approach in every person.

2. THERE IS NO BEST TREATMENT FOR EVERYONE WHO HAS A PARTICULAR TYPE OF ARTHRITIS, AS EACH INDIVIDUAL MAY RESPOND DIFFERENTLY TO DIFFERENT TREATMENTS.

In a chronic disease such as arthritis, there can be no best treatment for all people, because each person experiences his or her own individual set of symptoms and disease course. In addition, different people may experience very different responses to some of the drugs frequently used to treat arthritis. One person may find a particular medication to be extremely useful, while a second person may get no benefit at all from the same drug. A third might even have adverse effects from the drug and not be able to continue taking it. We hope you will always ask your health professional about new treatments and whether they might work for you. However, it's important to understand that there is no single best treatment for everyone.

3. NO SINGLE TYPE OF ARTHRITIS IS ALWAYS BETTER OR WORSE THAN ANOTHER TYPE.

Sometimes people ask, "Is rheumatoid arthritis worse than osteoarthritis?" or the other way around. It's true that, on average, some types of arthritis may cause more pain or disability than other types. However, arthritis affects each individual differently, and no type of arthritis is invariably better or worse than another type. For example, someone who has bursitis of the hip may experience more discomfort and functional disability than someone with a mild form of rheumatoid arthritis or osteoarthritis.

Some factors that contribute to the severity of the disease include: 1) how the condition affects daily life, including the ability to take care of yourself or continue to work; 2) how you react to symptoms of pain, fatigue, disability and psychological distress; and 3)

how you respond to treatments, including possible side effects. Any or all of these factors can affect how you – and the health professionals managing your care – perceive the severity of your arthritis.

4. INFORMATION FROM A PERSON WITH ARTHRITIS CAN BE AS VALUABLE IN DIAGNOSIS AND MANAGEMENT AS INFORMATION FROM LABORATORY TESTS AND X-RAYS.

In the traditional medical approach, doctors rely heavily on tests and data to diagnose and monitor a condition. These tests are often quite valuable in chronic diseases such as arthritis as well. But most important information is obtained directly from the person with arthritis. There is no single test that can diagnose or confirm most types of arthritis.

When talking to your doctor, *you* can provide the most important clues by answering the questions that are part of your patient history. In caring for chronically ill or debilitated people, doctors need to listen to more than just physical symptoms. Your doctor may also use a short questionnaire or diagram to get more information about your arthritis and how it affects your daily life and activities.

5. IN ARTHRITIS MANAGEMENT, THE EMPHASIS IS ON IMPROVING FUNCTION OF JOINTS AND RELIEVING PAIN.

The strategy in many illnesses is to try to get test measures, such as blood pressure, blood sugar (glucose) or cholesterol levels, back into the normal range. In contrast, strategies for managing rheumatic diseases are primarily to improve function, relieve pain, teach coping strategies and help people deal with the other associated problems seen in arthritis. Although the goals do include getting blood tests, such as an *elevated erythrocyte sedimentation rate (ESR or sed rate)* or *C-reactive protein (CRP)* into the normal range (see Chapter 4), the emphasis is on how you function from day to day. In general, it is just as important to focus on preserving and improving joint function and relieving pain, as on what laboratory tests or X-rays may reveal.

6. YOUR DOCTOR AND HEALTH-CARE TEAM NEED YOUR INVOLVEMENT IN ORDER TO HELP YOU TO THE FULLEST EXTENT. PEOPLE WITH ARTHRITIS AND HEALTH PROFESSIONALS ARE PARTNERS IN CARE.

If someone is acutely ill, the doctor may be expected to provide almost all the management, such as determining which tests are needed, selecting a treatment and administering these treatments. In a hospital, the doctor writes orders and treatments are provided by the hospital staff. The patient has no responsibility for treatment, other than cooperation.

Personally Speaking — Stories from real people with rheumatoid arthritis

"**B**efore rheumatoid arthritis started affecting the quality of my life, I enjoyed softball, basketball and walking. In 1995, at the age of 35, I was diagnosed with rheumatoid arthritis. It started out with little aches and pains, and taking pain relievers.

"By 1997, I was taking stronger medications and feeling my body changing. My hands, feet and knees were most affected, so I was discouraged from usual activities. After two years of inactivity, I was losing strength in my arms and legs, unable to grasp things or make a fist.

Swimming Saved My Life
by Janelle Peterson, Sonora, CA

"Desperate to improve my life, I tried swimming. First, I started with a water aerobics class. But jogging in place, part of the class's routine, bothered my feet.

"The Masters [seniors] swim class practiced right after the water aerobics class, so I stayed to watch them one day. I asked the coach if someone in my condition would be (challenged) in her class. She gave me a devilish grin and invited me to try her class.

"One year later, 25 pounds lighter, stronger, and nearly pain-free (with medication), I give thanks to this coach who motivates, inspires and encourages me to swim three to four times a week. Yes, life (mine) is great!"

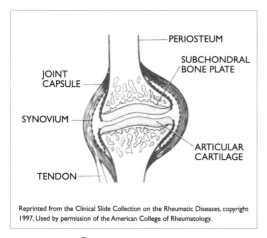

PERIOSTEUM

SUBCHONDRAL BONE PLATE

JOINT CAPSULE

SYNOVIUM

ARTICULAR CARTILAGE

TENDON

Reprinted from the Clinical Slide Collection on the Rheumatic Diseases, copyright 1997. Used by permission of the American College of Rheumatology.

DIAGRAM OF A HEALTHY JOINT

In a chronic disease, however, the doctor and health professionals can manage only a small component of the care. Professionals are certainly needed to guide diagnosis and treatment, but the patient is in control of the situation 99 percent of the time – spending less than a few hours each month or even each year with doctors and health professionals. A person with arthritis needs to be a very active participant in his or her care to get the best results.

Does this mean that you should not seek help from a doctor or other health professional? Of course not – but you and the health professionals you see should be partners in care. Many wonderful treatments are available to help people live well with arthritis. Decisions about treatments should not be considered orders, however; they should be viewed as cooperative arrangements between you and your health-care team. You – not the doctor or health professional – are ultimately in control of whether and when to take a medication, do exercises, practice good joint protection techniques or take any other steps toward controlling arthritis.

7. SOMETHING CAN ALWAYS BE DONE TO IMPROVE THE SITUATION FOR A PERSON WITH ARTHRITIS.

Old attitudes about arthritis suggested that "Arthritis is inevitable," or "Oh, it's arthritis – there's nothing you can do about it." On the contrary, there is *always* something that can be done to improve a situation for a person with arthritis. It may be a new drug, a device to make tasks easier, an exercise, a support group or maybe even a book like this one.

This is not to say that miracles exist. Instead, hard work on the part of the person with arthritis is usually needed to make things better. There are no cures yet. Most measures require some trade-offs in the form of time and effort spent on exercise, the cost of a new drug or device, or even mild medication side effects. However, you can be optimistic that your situation can be improved, because it always can!

Chapter 2

Rheumatoid Arthritis:

The Basics of a Chronic, Complex Disease

Rheumatoid arthritis (*def.*): A chronic disease in which inflammation of the joints (and sometimes other parts of the body) leads to long-term damage, which may result in chronic pain, loss of function and disability.

If you have rheumatoid arthritis, you've probably heard something similar to this definition from your doctor already. Perhaps you have wondered what all these terms mean. In this chapter, we're going to break down this definition into easily understood sections, and we hope to give you a better understanding of what happens in this complicated condition. We'll also give you some information about the history of rheumatoid arthritis, ongoing research into its possible causes and what it's like to have this disease.

Understanding Rheumatoid Arthritis

RHEUMATOID ARTHRITIS IS CHRONIC

Rheumatoid arthritis is considered a chronic disease because once it is established, it will continue relatively indefinitely and not go away. It can begin either suddenly or gradually. In some people with rheumatoid arthritis, particularly early in the disease, all signs of their arthritis gradually disappear. This is called a *spontaneous remission.*

If a spontaneous remission occurs, however, it is usually seen within six months of the onset of symptoms and swelling. If the pain and swelling continue for longer than six months, the problems are likely to become a persistent (chronic) condition.

Occasionally with rheumatoid arthritis, people may experience "attacks" of joint swelling that occur every few weeks or months, but then totally subside after only a few days. There may be no evidence of any arthritis between these attacks. This is known as *palindromic rheumatism.* (A palindrome is a phrase that reads the same forward and backward, such as "Madam I'm Adam.") About one half of people who experience palindromic rheumatism go on to develop chronic rheumatoid arthritis, with its characteristic persistent inflammation. Others continue to experience self-limited attacks for many years. In a lucky few, these attacks may even disappear.

Chronic diseases are best diagnosed and monitored using a patient-centered approach. In this approach, input from the person with arthritis is considered at least as, if not more, important as laboratory tests and values. Treatment is complex, usually involving a combination of drugs and other measures over time, rather than a single drug. And the person with the illness is a critical part of the disease-management team, using self-help measures, including mind-body approaches, to manage the disease day to day.

In fact, health professionals are generally "in control" of a person's chronic disease less than one-tenth of one percent of the time, or less than one hour per month. For the other 99.9 percent of the time, disease management is the responsibility of the person with the chronic illness. It is helpful to learn as much as you can about your particular disease, its course and treatment. You must become proactive in monitoring your symptoms and treatments and in handling the daily challenges your disease brings.

RHEUMATOID ARTHRITIS INVOLVES INFLAMMATION

When the body is threatened by some type of foreign invader, such as an infection, it normally mounts a response known as *inflammation* to help fight this threat. The chemicals released by the body to fight the infection cause a reaction that stimulates fever, swelling and associated pain, typical signs of inflammation.

In rheumatoid arthritis, inflammation of joints causes them to become swollen, tender and painful. Because inflammation in rheumatoid arthritis occurs throughout the body, organs other than joints – such as the eyes, lungs or others – may become involved in the process as well. People with rheumatoid arthritis often experience a flu-like illness, with fatigue and a poor sense of well-being.

For the most part, the early inflammatory process that occurs in the joints of people with rheumatoid arthritis is reversible. However, if unrecognized and untreated, uncontrolled inflammation – seen as chronic swelling and tenderness of joints – may lead to irreversible joint damage. Such damage can be documented on X-rays. Although each person experiences a different disease course, damage may begin as early as the first year of disease.

Joint damage caused by inadequately controlled inflammation ultimately leads to loss of joint movement, decreased ability to work, higher medical costs and potential surgery. It's very important to control the inflammation that occurs with rheumatoid arthritis as early and completely as possible with medications, as we will discuss later in this book.

RHEUMATOID ARTHRITIS INVOLVES AN ABNORMAL IMMUNE SYSTEM RESPONSE

Several types of white blood cells are involved in the immune response. One type of specialized white blood cell is known as a *B-lymphocyte*, a cell that produces *antibodies* directed to neutralize foreign substances known as *antigens*. These antibodies and antigens combine into what are known as "immune complexes," which are then removed by scavenger cells. Another class of cells are called T-lymphocytes, which regulate the function of B-cells by suppressing or stimulating the production of antibodies.

The immune system normally protects the body from disease through an elaborate network of signals that controls the production of antibodies when needed, and turns off this production when they are no longer needed. Normally, this elaborate control system works very well to maintain health. Under some circumstances, the signals do not function properly in people who develop rheumatoid arthritis. The immune system mistakenly thinks that the body itself is "foreign" rather than "self," a process known as *autoimmunity*. The immune cells then attack the body, causing inflammation that results in later damage to joints and other organs.

One interesting example of the incorrect signal referred to above is known as *rheumatoid factor*. Rheumatoid factor is an antibody that is directed to regulate normal antibodies made by an individual. Rheumatoid factor is a type of "anti-antibody," which may be normal in small quantities when the signals of the immune system function properly. However, excess amounts of rheumatoid factor may be seen when the signals do not function properly.

It is important to recognize that although rheumatoid factor is found in most people who have rheumatoid arthritis, it may not be found early in the disease. Furthermore, some people with severe rheumatoid arthritis never have rheumatoid factor. Even so, rheumatoid factor is a very important discovery in establishing that the immune system is incorrectly programmed in rheumatoid arthritis, leading to recent advances in treatments.

The immune system has been – and continues to be – the subject of much research. Many potential therapies for rheumatoid arthritis and other autoimmune diseases are targeted to "correcting" the faulty signals that distort the immune response, and/or to "overcoming" their consequences.

Who Gets Rheumatoid Arthritis?

It is estimated that rheumatoid arthritis affects about 0.5 percent to 1 percent of the population in the United States and most countries around the world. That's about 2.1 million Americans who have rheumatoid arthritis. Rheumatoid arthritis may begin at any age. It affects infants and the elderly, as well as those in the prime of life. More than 70 percent of people with rheumatoid arthritis are women, and the most common onset is between the ages of 40 and 50.

What Causes Rheumatoid Arthritis?

Although extensive research has been conducted throughout the 20th century, the cause (or causes) of rheumatoid arthritis remains unknown. Scientists have learned much about the immune response and the mechanisms of inflammation in arthritis (see the beginning of this chapter), but the actual triggering events that start the abnormal process are unknown.

Historically, rheumatoid arthritis was considered to be "chronic infectious arthritis," because its disease features were similar to those seen in infectious diseases like tuberculosis. Extensive efforts to identify a specific infectious agent (such as a bacterium, fungus or virus) that may cause rheumatoid arthritis have failed to pinpoint a culprit, however. More recently, researchers have tried to identify the "footprints" of an agent (such as the genetic material or DNA of an infectious agent) in the tissue of people with rheumatoid arthritis. To date, these studies remain inconclusive.

Even if a single infectious agent or footprints of such an agent were found consistently in people with rheumatoid arthritis, it is unlikely that everyone infected with this agent would get rheumatoid arthritis. The genetic makeup of an individual influences whether or not that individual develops an infection with any agent, even the common flu virus. Therefore, even if an infectious agent is found in most people with rheumatoid arthritis, the basis of why that person develops the disease would be explained only in part, with a need to look at other factors that contribute to the disease.

It is possible that what is now called rheumatoid arthritis actually includes many different diseases that are grouped together under the same name at this time. This has happened many times in the history of medicine. For instance, 150 years ago physicians recognized only one or a few types of pneumonia. Today, dozens of types of pneumonia have been described and categorized. Similarly, as more is learned about rheumatoid arthritis, many different diseases may be recognized as falling under the general umbrella of this condition.

THE ROLE OF GENDER

One important clue to the origin of rheumatoid arthritis is gender. As noted earlier, more than 70 percent of people with rheumatoid arthritis are women. This observation has led to theories that gender may play some part in the causation of rheumatoid arthritis and its severity.

Many women with rheumatoid arthritis experience improvement in their symptoms during pregnancy. Furthermore, rheumatoid arthritis develops more often than expected in the year after a pregnancy, and after a baby is born, women may experience an increase in symptoms. However, the understanding of possible effects of female hormones in rheumatoid arthritis remains limited at this time.

THE ROLE OF OTHER GENETIC FACTORS

In addition to gender, considerable progress has been made over the last 20 years in identifying specific genes that may be linked to an increased risk of developing rheumatoid arthritis. One such factor is known as the *major histocompatibility antigen*, which is found on the surface of lymphocytes and is known as *human lymphocyte antigen* (HLA). The HLA genetic site, or *locus*, controls immune responses. Researchers have shown that people with a specific genetic marker – known as the HLA shared epitope – were five times as likely to develop rheumatoid arthritis than people without the marker. More than two-thirds of Caucasian people with rheumatoid arthritis have this genetic marker, compared to only about 20 percent of the general population.

Although this genetic marker is associated with increased risk of disease and may be an important clue in the cause of rheumatoid arthritis, it cannot be used as a diagnostic test. This is because only a small minority of people with the shared epitope actually develop rheumatoid arthritis. In addition, many people with rheumatoid arthritis do not have this genetic marker.

Further research of genetic factors has led to the recognition that other yet-to-be-identified genes influence the development of

Personally Speaking — Stories from real people with rheumatoid arthritis

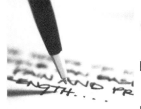

"**H**elp for arthritis comes in various forms, and not always from a prescription pad. My faithful dog and companion of 14 years, Freda, has helped me through some difficult times in dealing with arthritis.

"As a geriatric nurse practitioner, I realized that a therapy dog could be beneficial to elderly residents in the nursing home where I worked. In 1985, I purchased a bouncy fox terrier puppy. What positive changes I saw in the residents' moods!

A Four-Legged Prescription
by Linda Whitesell, Everett, WA

"In 1992, I experienced my first bout of rheumatoid arthritis. Freda was there for me, waiting patiently for the acute flares to subside so we could rejoin life. I remember how it hurt to pick up her ball to throw during our daily play time. She gave me hope and encouragement to stay active. After trials of different medications, we were finally back on track with our daily exercise routine.

"Our daily walks have become an important part of our therapy as Freda has developed arthritis, too. Even though our walks are slower, they are good 'medicine' for us. We both feel better, physically and emotionally. My pet is my friend and my therapist, helping me to keep going and enjoy life."

disease as well. One way in which researchers are continuing to search for these genes is by identifying families in which several members may have arthritis and analyzing their DNA (which makes up the genetic code).

NEW INSIGHTS

There have recently been new insights to suggest that stress may play a role in rheumatoid arthritis. A *stress* in this case can refer to a physical trauma, emotional upheaval or anything that stimulates the body to produce a stress response. Some researchers have suggested that rheumatoid arthritis may begin or worsen at times of stress.

In a normal stress response, the central nervous system responds to stress by sending out a complicated series of signals resulting in the production of corticosteroids by the body's adrenal glands. Thus, a stressful stimulus should lead to an increase in corticosteroid levels. Some people with rheumatoid arthritis appear to have a "blunted" response to stress, however, causing lower levels of corticosteroids to be produced. These observations may explain why people with rheumatoid arthritis often respond dramatically to small doses of drugs known as *glucocorticoids,* such as prednisone (see Chapter 11 on medications).

What Is It Like to Have Rheumatoid Arthritis?

Now that you've read all about the process of inflammation and what happens inside your body at a cellular level, what

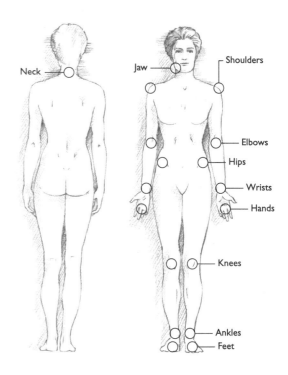

JOINTS THAT MAY BE AFFECTED BY RHEUMATOID ARTHRITIS

symptoms can you expect to experience from rheumatoid arthritis?

First of all, we must remember that each person is an individual, so the specific problems of one person with rheumatoid arthritis may differ substantially from those of another person with the same condition. Nonetheless, some problems are commonly seen in most people with rheumatoid arthritis, such as stiffness (especially in the morning), fatigue, and pain and swelling in many joints. While any joint may become involved, people commonly first experience symptoms of joint inflammation in the knuckles of the hands, the feet and the wrists. It is not uncommon for the elbows, shoulders, hips and knees to become involved as well.

A summary of the joints most likely to become involved in rheumatoid arthritis can be found in the illustration on page 14. The box on the right provides some key definitions that will help you understand the structure of your joints and how they are affected by inflammation.

In addition to these physical symptoms, people often experience psychological stress, frustration, helplessness and loss of control as they learn to cope with the day-to-day effects of a chronic disease. Psychological problems can, in turn, make it more difficult to cope with arthritis. Pain may even worsen. This cycle of pain can be helped through treatment and by developing skills – on your own or with the help of others – to cope with pain and psychological stress in positive, constructive ways.

Although arthritis is a chronic disease, many of the symptoms can be controlled – in fact, they *must* be controlled to prevent joint damage and disability. The good news is that the severe consequences seen in people with rheumatoid arthritis may now be prevented in most people. People with rheumatoid arthritis can feel more optimistic about their future than ever before. Drugs that are more effective and have fewer side effects than traditional medications are available now. These drugs are often used earlier in the disease, and in combination with one another, bringing about more effective control of inflammation. Exercise programs, joint protection activities

and a number of self-management techniques can significantly help people take control of their rheumatoid arthritis. All of these strategies will be discussed later in this book.

So, be informed, be proactive, but above all, be optimistic. You can learn to achieve good living with rheumatoid arthritis.

Your Joints: A Marvel of Engineering

A joint connects one bone to another. Joints come in various shapes and sizes: some move like a hinge (your finger and knee joints, for example); others have a "ball-in-socket" structure that allows them to move in many directions (your shoulder and hip joints); still others move in several different directions (your wrist and ankle). There are more than 70 movable joints in the human body, and rheumatoid arthritis can affect any of them.

Other soft-tissue structures surround the joint and may also be affected by arthritis. *Ligaments* are flexible bands of fibrous tissue that connect bones to one another. *Muscles* consist of fibers that stretch and tighten, allowing movement of the body's organs and joints. At the ends of muscles are the *tendons* that connect muscle to bone.

If you looked inside a joint, you would find *cartilage*, a smooth substance that lines the joint so your bones do not wear each other down. The *synovial fluid* found in the joint (the *synovium* is the lining of the joint) lubricates it and allows free movement. When joints are actively inflamed, inflammatory cells are found in the synovial fluid and synovial lining, and cause breakdown of cartilage and bone.

Chapter 3

Diagnostic Methods

Your Medical History and Physical Examination

Whether you've had rheumatoid arthritis for a while, or you've only begun to suspect that you may have it, you probably want to know more about how your doctor diagnoses this condition. This chapter and the one that follows will try to shed some light on the processes that doctors use to determine whether you have rheumatoid arthritis. The more you know about these methods — and the importance of the information you can provide — the better you will become at understanding and participating in the process.

There is currently no laboratory test that can absolutely determine whether or not you have rheumatoid arthritis. In this way, the diagnosis differs from other diseases, such as diabetes or kidney failure, in which very specific and simple blood tests can confirm the diagnoses in most people. By contrast, the rheumatoid factor (the antibody discussed in the previous chapter whose presence may indicate rheumatoid arthritis) test is positive in many people with rheumatoid arthritis, but is negative in 20 percent to 30 percent of the people who have this disease. Furthermore, a test for rheumatoid factor may be positive in people who do not have rheumatoid arthritis.

Even discovering which kind of arthritis a person has is not always easy. As we discussed in Chapter 1, each person experiences his or her own individual disease course, and a person may have more than one type of rheumatic condition. A skilled physician will use the information provided by the patient and the findings of a physical examination to decide a likely diagnosis and determine which tests are needed. In fact, the most important parts of the diagnostic process are a careful medical history, including a full discussion of symptoms, and a complete physical exam.

This chapter will discuss the components of your medical history and physical examination. The chapter that follows will discuss some of the more commonly used tests for helping to diagnose rheumatoid arthritis, in addition to explaining why these tests do not always provide a clear answer to the question: Do I have rheumatoid arthritis?

The "Low-Tech" Tools

It should be no surprise to you that the practice of medicine has become very "high tech" throughout the latter part of the 20th century. Batteries of tests and the use of expensive imaging equipment have become standard. However, in rheumatoid arthritis, the most important and perhaps surprising tools for diagnosis are the "low-tech" components of your office visit – your medical history and physical examination.

MEDICAL HISTORY

Ever wonder why you have to fill out forms and answer so many questions when you visit your doctor? No, it's not just a plot to keep you busy while you wait – you are actually providing much of the information your doctor needs to make a diagnosis of rheumatoid arthritis. There are many diagnostic clues in the answers you supply during the medical history part of your office visit. Some of the key questions that you may be asked include the following:

• **Do you have joint pain in many joints?** People who have rheumatoid arthritis usually experience joint involvement in several joints at once, as opposed to having pain in only one joint.

• **Does the pain occur symmetrically – that is, do the same joints on both sides of your body hurt at the same time? Or is the pain one-sided?** Symmetric pain is often a sign of rheumatoid arthritis. For instance, if both wrists are swollen, or the same knuckles in both hands, rheumatoid arthritis may be a possibility.

• **Do you have stiffness in the morning?** Morning stiffness, another hallmark of rheumatoid arthritis, occurs when the joints feel stiff and are difficult to move. Doctors are often interested in how long your morning stiffness lasts. After a period of loosening up, motion becomes easier and less painful. Stiffness is likely to recur after sitting for prolonged periods of time.

• **When is the pain most severe?** For example, do your joints hurt more in the morning or late in the day? Inflammation, like that seen in rheumatoid arthritis, often is associated with joints feeling better with moderate activity, but greater discomfort may occur in the early morning and later in the day, when fatigue sets in.

• **Do you have pain in your hands, wrists and/or feet?** Although rheumatoid arthritis can occur in any joint of the body, these joints are most frequently involved and cause symptoms of pain and swelling.

• **If you have pain in your hands, which joints hurt the most?** In rheumatoid arthritis, rows of joints such as those where your fingers make their first bend (metacarpophalangeal joints) and the middle knuckles of the fingers (proximal interphalangeal joints) tend to be affected more often than the knuckles near the tips of the fingers.

• **Have you had periods of feeling weak and uncomfortable all over? Do you feel fatigued?** Many people with rheumatoid arthritis notice generalized problems, such as muscle aches, fatigue, stiffness, weight loss and a general "flu-like" feeling.

Your answers to these and other questions often let the doctor know if rheumatoid arthritis should be considered as a diagnosis.

And, if you have already been diagnosed with rheumatoid arthritis, your medical history will continue to play a starring role in your office visits, as your doctor will want to keep close tabs on your pain and functional status, any developing limitations in your abilities to perform activities, your medications, and any side effects you may experience.

PATIENT QUESTIONNAIRES

Patient self-report questionnaires, in addition to the medical history, are increasingly

---

Personally Speaking Stories from real people with rheumatoid arthritis

"When I was first diagnosed with rheumatoid arthritis, my primary problems were learning to deal with the pain and the frustration of not being able to continue my active lifestyle.

"After trying several medications, even participating in two clinical drug trials, I showed little major improvement. I realized it was up to me to find ways to cope with the disease on a daily basis.

Six Keys to Coping: Staying Busy and Interested in Life
by Nancy Block,
Irving, TX

"These are six strategies that have helped me deal with rheumatoid arthritis:

• Planning ahead and allowing plenty of time for an activity or project.
• Staying busy and involved with other people.
• Appreciating what I am able to do each day.
• Learning that it is all right to say no to activities that would be too difficult or stressful, and not feeling guilty about it.
• Listening to music with headphones. With no outside distractions, I can focus on the healing power of music instead of the pain.
• Going back to college after 30 years. Concentrating on something other than pain, learning new things, making new friends, and obtaining my associate's degree at the same time.

"This disease is a major part of my life. By staying busy and interested in the world around me, the pain is lessened and I am able to accomplish more every day."

used by doctors to provide critical information about your disease course and treatment. Some of the most important problems experienced by people with rheumatoid arthritis, including loss of function, pain, fatigue and psychological distress, are not measured directly by any blood test, X-ray or other high-tech measure. Doctors use the results from patient questionnaires to assess the impact of rheumatoid arthritis on daily life.

If your doctor is not currently using a patient questionnaire, you may want to consider discussing it with him or her, because these measures have been proven to be one of the most effective ways to monitor changes in disease over a five- to 10-year period. Several self-report questionnaires have been tested and widely used in the care of people with rheumatoid arthritis. Two of the most common are described below.

• **The Health Assessment Questionnaire (HAQ).** This measurement tool includes 20 activities of daily living in eight categories including dressing, eating, walking and other activities. Participants are also asked to measure their pain and their overall outlook, and to answer questions about their use of aids and devices. Modified versions (modified HAQ, and multidimensional HAQ) have been developed to provide additional data within a two-page format that includes global status, measures of fatigue and psychological distress, and medication review.

• **The Arthritis Impact Measurement Scales (AIMS).** This tool includes several dimensions of health status including mobility, physical activity, dexterity, household activities, anxiety, depression and social activities, in addition to activities of daily living and pain.

PHYSICAL EXAMINATION

After your medical history, a thorough physical examination by a doctor knowledgeable about rheumatoid arthritis will usually supply most of the necessary information to make a diagnosis. The doctor will look for the features commonly seen in this chronic condition, which may include any of the following:

• **Joint swelling.** This may be severe or barely noticeable. A skilled doctor should be able to recognize even slight joint swelling that may indicate rheumatoid arthritis.

• **Joint tenderness.** Certain joints may be painful to even the slightest touch.

• **Loss of motion in your joints.** This may indicate inflammation (see Chapter 2 for a description of the inflammatory process) or joint damage. The physician will assess your joints' range of motion. For instance, can you move your shoulders through a complete circle?

• **Joint malalignment.** After several years of rheumatoid arthritis (especially if inflammation is unchecked), some joint damage often occurs, causing joints to be out of alignment. This is most commonly seen in the small joints of the hands and feet.

• **Signs of rheumatoid arthritis in other organs.** Rheumatoid arthritis is a *systemic* disease, meaning it may affect other systems in your body. The doctor will look for involvement in other parts of the body including your skin, lungs and eyes, among others.

The doctor will review each joint during the physical exam to determine which joints have signs of arthritis, including tenderness, pain on motion, swelling, limited motion and long-term damage. *Joint counts* have been shown to be quite useful to assess, monitor and predict the course of rheuma-

toid arthritis in individuals. Usually, your doctor will not only make a complete count of which joints are involved, but also will assess the severity of the involvement in each joint.

PHYSICAL MEASURES OF FUNCTION

Your doctor may want to get an idea of your ability to perform certain tasks. Physical function measures may indicate both evidence of inflammation and evidence of long-term damage. They may be done by someone in a doctor's office or by a physical or occupational therapist. Some widely used measures include the following:

• **Grip strength.** The traditional method for measuring grip strength has been to inflate a blood pressure cuff and ask the individual to squeeze as hard as possible, first with the right then with the left hand. The pressure change on the cuff is recorded. The test is usually repeated several times.
• **Walking time.** The individual is asked to walk a set distance (usually 25 or 50 feet) at a normal pace. The time to complete the distance is then recorded.
• **Button test.** The individual is asked to unbutton and button five buttons as quickly as possible using a standard button board. The score is recorded in seconds.

CLASSIFICATION CRITERIA

You may have heard or read about something called "classification criteria for rheumatoid arthritis" (see box, left). These

---

Classification Criteria for Rheumatoid Arthritis

These very specific classification criteria were developed by members of the American College of Rheumatology. The criteria describe patterns of symptoms that are most commonly seen in people with rheumatoid arthritis. They can be used as guidelines, but they will not give you or your doctor specific information about your prognosis (what will happen over time with your condition).

Classification Criteria
1. Morning stiffness
2. Arthritis of three or more joints
3. Arthritis of more than two hand joints
4. Symmetrical arthritis
5. Subcutaneous (rheumatoid) nodules
6. Rheumatoid factor
7. Radiographic (X-ray) changes

Adapted from Revised Classification Criteria for Rheumatoid Arthritis, *Arthritis and Rheumatism*, 1988, Volume 31, pp. 315-324, by Arnett, Edworthy, Bloch, et al.

criteria were developed by a committee of rheumatologists (doctors who specialize in treating arthritis) and provide a guideline to the patterns of findings usually seen in rheumatoid arthritis.

Summary

As you can see, your doctor is able to obtain most of the valuable information needed to make a diagnosis of rheumatoid arthritis before a laboratory test is ever ordered. Your contribution can be substan-tial by providing clear and accurate information on your own medical history, as well as any family history of arthritis or joint symptoms. It is also a good idea to keep track of which joints have been swollen or painful, because the disease may abate in some joints and flare in others over time.

Having said this, there is a place in the diagnosis of rheumatoid arthritis for certain laboratory tests that provide additional information to your doctor. These tests are discussed in the next chapter.

Chapter 4

Diagnosing
Rheumatoid Arthritis:

Laboratory Tests and Imaging Studies

Like the pieces of a puzzle, the information and clues that you and your doctor uncover will fit together in a way that will help determine whether or not you have rheumatoid arthritis. As you may already know from previous chapters, there is currently no laboratory test that can *absolutely* determine whether or not you have rheumatoid arthritis.

People with rheumatoid arthritis can have normal test results, and people can have abnormal test results yet not have rheumatoid arthritis. *As a result, the interpretation of laboratory tests depends on the symptoms of the individual.* This is why the information provided by you and discovered during the physical examination is so crucial to the diagnosis. Tests are widely used by physicians because they can add certainty to a diagnosis, when combined with information provided by a patient.

This chapter discusses several tests used to help diagnose rheumatoid arthritis. Some of the tests may be familiar to you. Others are used less commonly and may not be necessary for you. You may feel that you are looking into a bowl of alphabet soup as you ponder the importance of your ESR, RF, ANA and MRI, among others. But all of these tests can provide important clues when used in the right way.

When These Tests Are Helpful

Laboratory tests and imaging procedures can be helpful because they may be used to confirm the doctor's diagnosis. In addition, they may help determine the severity of disease activity.

There is a long list of laboratory tests and imaging studies that may be used to help diagnose rheumatoid arthritis. For any one person, however, only a few such tests may be needed. Some of the most commonly used laboratory measures are explained in this section.

Be aware that your doctor may choose to order only one or two tests, or he or she may use a test not described here. In general, tests used for diagnosis do not need to be repeated after the diagnosis is made. Other tests, designed to check for drug side effects or to measure improvement, may need to be repeated at regular intervals.

Laboratory Tests Used in Diagnosis

COMPLETE BLOOD COUNT

Counts of different types of blood cells are used in the assessment of patients with many types of diseases. There are three cellular components of blood: red blood cells carry oxygen to tissues, white blood cells help the body fight infections, and platelets are needed to stop bleeding and form clots.

Measurement of these cells is often done during the first office visit and may be repeated during treatment to monitor for possible side effects from drugs and sometimes to check progress in reversing abnormalities.

Red blood cells are evaluated according to measures of hemoglobin, hematocrit and a red blood cell count. *Hemoglobin* is the protein in red blood cells that carries oxygen from the lungs to the tissues; it may be low in rheumatoid arthritis because of the "anemia of chronic disease." Similarly, the *hematocrit* (which measures the volume of red blood cells) and the red blood cell count (which measures the number of red blood cells) may be lower than normal in people with rheumatoid arthritis. The anemia seen in people with rheumatoid arthritis may contribute to feelings of fatigue or malaise. People with more aggressive disease tend to have more severe anemia.

White blood cells may also be counted. A high count may mean that an infection is present and can be a sign of severe inflammation. However, the white blood cell count is usually normal in people with rheumatoid arthritis, unless a simultaneous infection is present. (The white cell count may be low in an unusual complication of rheumatoid arthritis called Felty's syndrome, which is discussed later.) Some of the medications used to treat rheumatoid arthritis may cause a reduction in the white cell count, thereby reducing the body's capacity to fight infections. This is why the white blood cell count is monitored periodically in people with rheumatoid arthritis.

Platelets are small cells that participate in the formation of blood clots. The platelet count may be elevated when inflammation is severe, or it may be depressed (lowered) by certain drugs. The platelet count and the white blood cell count are monitored about every six months in people who take only nonsteroidal anti-inflammatory drugs (NSAIDs), such as ibuprofen and naproxen, and about every two to 12 weeks in people who take most disease-modifying antirheumatic drugs (DMARDs), such as methotrexate and leflunomide.

ERYTHROCYTE SEDIMENTATION RATE

The erythrocyte sedimentation rate (which your doctor may call your ESR or sed rate) is a valuable test often used to assess the degree of inflammation. The test is a measurement of how fast red blood cells (erythrocytes) fall to the bottom of a glass tube that is filled with blood and allowed to sit for one hour. People with any type of inflammation, including rheumatoid arthritis, often have higher sedimentation rates than those in the normal range. If the level of inflammation is reduced with treatment, the sedimentation rate usually drops. Because it is so important to control inflammation in rheumatoid arthritis, this test may be repeated fairly frequently.

One problem is that the ESR is elevated in only about 60 percent of people who have rheumatoid arthritis – meaning that the remaining 40 percent have a normal sedimentation rate. Remember: The primary basis for your treatment is generally directed by the severity of your clinical symptoms, such as pain and functional ability. Therefore, even if your ESR is normal, treatment for your rheumatoid arthritis often should continue.

C-REACTIVE PROTEIN

C-reactive protein (or CRP) is another substance found in the body that indicates the presence of inflammation. Elevated levels of this protein provide an additional measure of disease activity in rheumatoid arthritis. Although the ESR and CRP often reflect similar degrees of inflammation, sometimes ESR levels are elevated when CRP levels are normal (and vice versa). This phenomenon is not well understood.

Some researchers have recognized that CRP levels that remain high over a long period are often associated with more severe joint damage later in the disease. This pro-

vides a strong rationale for trying to reduce the CRP to normal levels. However, some people with normal levels of CRP may still experience progressive joint damage.

As with the sedimentation rate, treatment for rheumatoid arthritis usually should continue even if CRP levels are normal. This test may be repeated at regular intervals to monitor the level of inflammation and your response to medication.

RHEUMATOID FACTOR

Some abnormal *antibodies* (special proteins produced by B-lymphocytes of the immune system in response to substances such as infectious agents) are often found in the blood of people with rheumatoid arthritis that are not commonly found in people without the disease.

Rheumatoid factor (RF) is an antibody found in the blood of about 70 percent to 80 percent of people with rheumatoid arthritis. It is found in the serum component of the blood – the other half of the blood from the cellular components discussed above as red blood cells, white blood cells and platelets. It is an antibody directed to neutralize normal antibodies, as discussed in Chapter 2. These antibodies are normally produced by the body and are known as gamma globulins or immunoglobulin G (IgG).

Most people with rheumatoid arthritis have a large amount of rheumatoid factor circulating in the blood. However, the rheumatoid factor test is not a specific diagnostic test for rheumatoid arthritis. At least one in five people with rheumatoid arthritis does not have rheumatoid factor, but does have a form of the disease that cannot be distinguished from people who have rheumatoid factor.

People with rheumatoid arthritis who do not have rheumatoid factor in their blood or serum are often referred to as "seronegative." As noted, their disease doesn't differ from that of "seropositive" people who have rheumatoid factor in their serum. The rheumatoid factor test, also called the rheumatoid arthritis latex test, measures the amount of these antibodies in *titers* or units. A titer is simply a number to indicate the dilution of blood at which rheumatoid factor may be detected, so that if the titer is 1:160, there is twice as much rheumatoid factor as if the titer is 1:80. Rheumatoid factor may also be measured in units: higher numbers mean more rheumatoid factor. However, test results may be negative during the first several months, making this test less useful in early diagnosis of rheumatoid arthritis. But, over time, this test for rheumatoid factor is positive in 60 percent to 80 percent of people with rheumatoid arthritis.

It was once thought that people who had a positive rheumatoid factor test were more likely to have a severe disease course. Recent studies suggest that the differences in disease severity between those who do and do not have rheumatoid factor are not necessarily as great as researchers once believed.

ANTINUCLEAR ANTIBODIES

Another test for abnormal antibodies is called the antinuclear antibody (ANA) test.

It detects a group of *autoantibodies* (antibodies against self) that combine with the nuclei of cells. These particular antibodies are most often positive in people with systemic lupus erythematosus, but they are also seen in about 30 percent to 40 percent of people with rheumatoid arthritis. In addition, a positive ANA test may be seen in people with scleroderma (systemic sclerosis), polymyositis and other inflammatory rheumatic diseases.

It is important to be aware that most people with positive antinuclear antibody tests have neither rheumatoid arthritis nor lupus, and probably have no disease at all. Because of the difficulty of interpreting meaningful results, many doctors no longer routinely use this test in diagnosing rheumatoid arthritis.

GENETIC TYPING

In recent years, much attention has been focused on the search for genetic markers that may predispose certain people to develop (or be susceptible to) a particular disease. About two-thirds of people with rheumatoid arthritis have a genetic marker known as a *shared epitope* at the major histocompatibility locus (see Chapter 2), or the area where the genes that control the immune system response are located.

Although identification of this shared epitope is critical for research studies to understand how rheumatoid arthritis develops, we must recognize that about seven percent of the normal population have the shared epitope but do not develop rheumatoid arthritis.

Furthermore, at least 20 percent of those with rheumatoid arthritis do not have the shared epitope. Measurement of the epitope is not useful in diagnosing rheumatoid arthritis, because it will often give incorrect impressions.

URINALYSIS

A routine study done on the urine (urinalysis or UA) includes tests for sugar (which can identify and monitor diabetes), protein (seen when kidney abnormalities are present) or abnormal cells that indicate inflammation or infection of the kidney, bladder or other parts of the urinary tract. A urinalysis is not helpful in the diagnosis of rheumatoid arthritis, but it is used regularly in people with rheumatoid arthritis who are treated with certain medications such as gold or penicillamine (see chapter 11). These drugs may cause damage to the kidneys in a few patients, so monitoring is necessary.

Imaging Studies
RADIOGRAPHS (X-RAYS)

X-rays taken early in the course of rheumatoid arthritis can show swelling of the soft tis-

---

Personally Speaking Stories from real people with rheumatoid arthritis

"I am a 61-year-old with severe rheumatoid arthritis. My hands are drawn, I have fused wrists, a fused neck, deformed joints in my feet. But I am active, and on the go most of the time.

"I developed rheumatoid arthritis at 18. Quickly, I saw that I was going to have to learn all I could about this thing that was so rapidly changing my life, in order to be able to cope with it. I prayed to God to help me be as normal as I could be around my family and friends, and to help me with the pain.

Don't Let 'Arthur' Take Charge
by Carlyn Creel, Weaver, AL

"I talk to my family about my problems, but I don't give a daily account of every pain. My husband will sometimes say, 'You are having a rough day, aren't you?' And I say, 'Arthur thinks he is in charge today – but he is not!'

"Once, when I was depressed about my pain and how I looked, my niece who had cancer called, telling me about her chemotherapy and her concern about losing her hair. Her call changed my attitude. I wondered why I was feeling so sorry for myself. She was fighting for her life, and I was not. I needed to help her!

"If I see someone staring at me in public, I smile at them, and I always get a big smile back. About 50 percent of coping is your mental attitude. It's like a daily ride on a roller coaster, with ups and downs. But you can still have fun and joy in your life."

sues and loss of bone density around the joints because of the patient's reduced activity and inflammation. In later disease, about 70 percent of people with rheumatoid arthritis will develop *erosions* (small holes) near the ends of bones and narrowing of the joint space due to loss of cartilage.

Doctors once thought that because of the potential side effects, aggressive drug treatment should not be given until erosions were seen, to be sure that someone who receives such treatment has rheumatoid arthritis. It is now widely recognized that it is best to treat aggressively and early before there is damage to joints caused by erosions. X-rays are not necessarily used as guides to initiate treatment, but they remain important in evaluating how well certain treatments may control joint damage, and to help recognize when people may be candidates for joint surgery.

X-rays taken early in the disease course can provide a valuable baseline for comparison with later X-rays to see if and how the disease may progress. Many authorities have proposed that people with rheumatoid arthritis should have routine X-rays of the hands and feet every one to two years.

BONE SCANS

Bone scans may be used to detect evidence of inflammation in the body, including joints. While bone scans may be used to confirm the presence of *polyarthritis* (arthritis affecting multiple joints), this can usually be detected in a physical examination. Bone scans are gen-erally not necessary to make a diagnosis of rheumatoid arthritis.

MAGNETIC RESONANCE IMAGING (MRI)

An MRI scan can detect early inflammation before X-ray changes are seen. These scans are effective at pinpointing *synovitis* (inflammation of the lining of the joint) in many people who show no damage on X-rays. It is possible that over the next few years MRI scanning will become an important diagnostic aid and method for monitoring the degree of arthritis activity in a joint or joints.

JOINT ULTRASOUND

Joint ultrasound is a much less expensive way to look for joint inflammation before X-rays show damage. Although not currently used often, this procedure may gain wider use over the next few years as doctors increase their efforts to document early evidence of disease.

BONE DENSITOMETRY

Bone densitometry is an important imaging study for measuring bone density, used primarily to detect *osteoporosis*, a major clinical problem for older people, particularly women. Osteoporosis may be especially severe in people with rheumatoid arthritis due to joint immobilization, the inflammatory response itself, and the use of certain therapies (such as glucocorticoids) that may hasten bone loss. Some doctors suggest that a bone density test should be part of the evaluation and monitoring of all people with rheumatoid arthritis, particularly for women after menopause.

Chapter 5

Diagnosis
Checkpoints:

What if It's *not* Rheumatoid Arthritis?

For the majority of people with rheumatoid arthritis, establishing a diagnosis can be done with confidence. But even skilled rheumatologists on occasion may have difficulty determining whether a person has rheumatoid arthritis or one of several other diseases that can have similar symptoms.

To further muddy the waters, when large groups of patients are studied over long periods of time, about five percent of people who were originally diagnosed as having rheumatoid arthritis actually turn out to have another type of rheumatic disease five to 10 years later. Another five percent of people who were thought to have other rheumatic diseases may turn out to have rheumatoid arthritis.

What is recognized today as the single disease "rheumatoid arthritis" probably involves many different types of diseases (see Chapter 2). In the future, physicians may well be able to distinguish several different forms of rheumatoid arthritis. This may partly explain why a diagnosis of rheumatoid arthritis can be associated with such variation in the number of joints or organs affected, the severity of symptoms, and the way the disease responds to therapy.

In this chapter, we take a look at some of the many other types of rheumatic diseases whose symptoms can sometimes mimic or resemble rheumatoid arthritis (see the box).

Diseases That Can Resemble Rheumatoid Arthritis
Osteoarthritis *
Fibromyalgia*
Gout
Ankylosing spondylitis
Bursitis and Tendinitis*
Sjögren's syndrome*
Felty's syndrome *
Connective Tissue Diseases:
Systemic lupus erythematosus (lupus)
Scleroderma
Polymyositis/Dermatomyositis
Vasculitis

* indicates disease/syndromes that may occur commonly together with rheumatoid arthritis.

Some of these diseases can even occur together with rheumatoid arthritis, making it even more important to obtain an accurate diagnosis and determine appropriate treatment.

Osteoarthritis

Osteoarthritis (sometimes called degenerative joint disease) occurs when joint cartilage is worn away, causing damage and eventual destruction of the joint. This condition was once thought to be an inevitable part of getting old, and certainly the chance of developing it increases with age. However, many people never develop osteoarthritis, and many people with osteoarthritis do not show any progression over five to 10 years. New research suggests that active mechanisms – not just the process of aging – play a part in the development of osteoarthritis.

It is usually a simple matter to distinguish between osteoarthritis and rheumatoid arthritis. There are forms of osteoarthritis, however, that can look deceptively like rheumatoid arthritis. One such form is *erosive osteoarthritis*, in which the middle knuckle joints and/or the knuckles closest to the tips of the fingers often show bony enlargement. On X-rays, erosions are seen that can look very much like those seen in rheumatoid arthritis. The knuckles nearest the wrist are generally *not* involved in erosive osteoarthritis, which provides one way to distinguish this form of osteoarthritis from rheumatoid arthritis. The wrists, elbows and ankles also are generally not involved in erosive osteoarthritis, but are joints commonly affected in rheumatoid arthritis.

Occasionally, people develop osteoarthritis that is *symmetric* (affects the same joints on both sides of the body), which is a hallmark of rheumatoid arthritis. This may be seen primarily as involvement of both hands, hips or knees.

Sometimes when a joint already has extensive damage from the inflammatory process of rheumatoid arthritis, but the inflammation itself is no longer present, the doctor may not be sure whether the damage was caused by osteoarthritis or rheumatoid arthritis. A detailed patient history and examination of other joints will usually

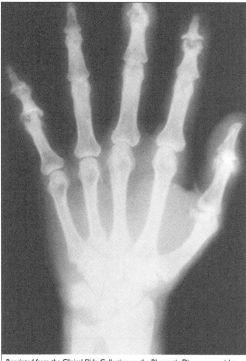

Reprinted from the Clinical Slide Collection on the Rheumatic Diseases, copyright 1997. Used by permission of the American College of Rheumatology.

EROSIVE OSTEOARTHRITIS

allow the physician to determine the cause of the damage. At this point, the cause of damage is less important than addressing the damage itself (for instance, through the need for joint replacement surgery).

Fibromyalgia

Fibromyalgia is a syndrome that, like rheumatoid arthritis, is more common among women. About 90 percent of people with fibromyalgia are women, compared with 70 percent of people with rheumatoid arthritis. The most common symptom is widespread, generalized musculoskeletal pain, which may occur in the back, shoulders, neck or any other part of the body. This widespread pain may raise a concern that the patient has rheumatoid arthritis, but there is no joint swelling or other evidence of inflammation in the joints seen in fibromyalgia.

People with fibromyalgia often have a history of sleep difficulties, and they may also experience problems in other organ systems – such as migraine headaches or irritable bowel syndrome. These problems are not associated with damage to the body, but can cause severe distress.

Although people with fibromyalgia may experience joint tenderness, this sensitivity is usually generalized to muscle groups. However, people with rheumatoid arthritis may also not have joint swelling at times during the course of their disease, and they

Disease Differences

Osteoarthritis	Rheumatoid Arthritis
Usually begins after age 40	Usually begins between ages 15 and 50
Usually develops slowly, over many years	May develop suddenly, within weeks or months
Affects a few joints and may occur on both sides of the body	Usually affects many joints, primarily the small joints on both sides of the body
Joint redness, warmth and swelling is usually minimal. Morning stiffness is common and may be severe but brief	Causes redness, warmth, swelling and prolonged morning stiffness of the joints
Affects only certain joints; rarely affects wrists, elbows or ankles	Affects many joints including wrists, elbows and shoulders
Doesn't cause a general feeling of sickness and fatigue	Often causes a general feeling of sickness and fatigue, as well as weight loss and fever

may show evidence of fibromyalgia. It appears that fibromyalgia is considerably more common in people with rheumatoid arthritis than in the general population – and in fact, some people have both rheumatoid arthritis and fibromyalgia. When this happens, both conditions may be mild, or one may be mild and the other severe.

It is important to distinguish whether rheumatoid arthritis or fibromyalgia may account for symptoms, because drugs used to treat rheumatoid arthritis usually do not help the symptoms that result from fibromyalgia. However, because many symptoms are common in both rheumatoid arthritis and fibromyalgia, including generalized muscle pain, morning stiffness, difficulty sleeping soundly and fatigue, the doctor and patient must sometimes make an educated guess about the likely cause of particular symptoms.

Gout

Gout has been called "the great masquerader" because it can mimic almost any other rheumatic disease. Gout occurs when an excess of *uric acid* in the body leads to the formation of crystals in the joint. The crystals then stimulate an inflammatory response that can cause an extremely painful episode or attack of arthritis. Although gout most often occurs in the big toe, called *podagra,* it can involve virtually any joint or joints and, in time, the attacks may become chronic and may resemble rheumatoid arthritis.

Certain features help distinguish gout from rheumatoid arthritis. First, gout usually occurs in men, while rheumatoid arthritis is more common in women. Second, gout usually does not involve the hands (at least in early disease), but rheumatoid arthritis does. Third, most discomfort in gout occurs episodically, rather than continually as in rheumatoid arthritis.

It is important to distinguish between gout and rheumatoid arthritis because there are specific medications that can lower uric acid levels and control gout attacks. Different drugs are used to control the inflammation seen in rheumatoid arthritis.

Ankylosing Spondylitis

Ankylosing spondylitis is another generalized form of arthritis that can resemble rheumatoid arthritis. The joints commonly involved in ankylosing spondylitis are in the back, neck and in large joints such as the shoulders, hips and knees. This differs from rheumatoid arthritis, which tends to affect the small joints of the hands and feet. As with gout, ankylosing spondylitis is thought to be more common among men, while rheumatoid arthritis is seen more often in women. Nevertheless, women also develop ankylosing spondylitis.

Although ankylosing spondylitis is a systemic disease like rheumatoid arthritis, it does not usually cause as much fatigue or a poor sense of well-being.

The inflammation in ankylosing spondylitis occurs in the *enthesis,* or the place where the tendon inserts into the bone, as well as in the lining of the joint as seen in rheumatoid arthritis. Perhaps because of this, people with ankylosing spondylitis tend to respond to different drugs, as well as different types of exercise programs. These treatment differences reinforce the importance of correct diagnosis.

Researchers have located a genetic marker (known as HLA-B27) that is associated with ankylosing spondylitis, reminiscent of the shared epitope of rheumatoid arthritis. However, this genetic marker is not a good diagnostic test for the disease because most people with the HLA-B27 marker do not have ankylosing spondylitis.

Some studies suggest that women with ankylosing spondylitis are more likely to experience signs of generalized inflammation – including more fatigue, a poor sense of well-being and joint swelling – than men with ankylosing spondylitis.

Bursitis and Tendinitis

Bursitis and tendinitis are common conditions known as soft tissue rheumatic syndromes. They are characterized by pain and inflammation in the structures and tissues around the joints. Bursitis is an irritation or inflammation of the *bursa*, a small sac located between bone and muscle, skin or tendon that allows for smooth movement between these structures. Tendinitis is an irritation or inflammation of the tendon, a cord that attaches muscle to bone.

The pain of bursitis and tendinitis are located near joints, so some people may mistake this pain for that of arthritis. But arthritis is the inflammation of the joint itself, not the structures around the joint.

Sjögren's Syndrome

Sjögren's syndrome, which is also called sicca ("dry") syndrome, involves the salivary

Checkpoint: Your Diagnosis

Rheumatoid arthritis is not just the aches and pains of aging or of old injuries. It is a serious chronic illness that can affect many organs in your body. If you think you may have rheumatoid arthritis, you should see your doctor as soon as possible. Please remember that laboratory testing can be helpful, but does not provide the definitive information to make a diagnosis.

Not all doctors have extensive experience in the diagnosis and treatment of rheumatoid arthritis. You should get a second opinion from a rheumatologist – a specialist in rheumatoid arthritis and related conditions. It is very important to control the joint inflammation of rheumatoid arthritis as early and as effectively as possible. This reduces the chance of permanent damage and disability from rheumatoid arthritis.

Remember, you are the most important member of your health-care team, but you can't do it alone. Play it safe and see a doctor.

and lacrimal (tear-producing) glands, leading to dry eyes and dry mouth. About 30 percent of people with rheumatoid arthritis have some evidence of Sjögren's syndrome.

Sjögren's syndrome is often diagnosed through a medical history and physical examination. Some doctors may also use any of a variety of tests. These tests may include a blood test to check the level of certain antibodies; tests to measure the dryness of eyes; a lip biopsy to examine the salivary glands; a salivary function test; or a urine test to check kidney function.

Your doctor may send you to an ophthalmologist, an eye specialist, for an eye examination and to conduct some tests.

Sjögren's syndrome may be treated by a number of medications. Simple self-management strategies are also helpful, such as sipping water or chewing sugar-free gum or candies to temporarily ease dry mouth, and using over-the-counter lubricating eye drops to relieve dry eyes.

Felty's Syndrome

Felty's syndrome is a form of rheumatoid arthritis in which there is an enlargement of the spleen and a reduced number of white blood cells. Patients with Felty's syndrome are at increased risk for the development of infections. In some cases, it may be regarded (and treated) as a more severe form of rheumatoid arthritis.

Aggressive treatment with gold salts or methotrexate may be effective, even though they may not seem appropriate initially because they may reduce the white blood cell count. Sometimes

When Your Doctor Isn't Sure

Despite a medical history, physical examination and the appropriate tests, your doctor still isn't 100 percent sure whether you have rheumatoid arthritis or another type of inflammatory rheumatic disease. How worried should you be?

Well, you can relax a bit. By tracking many people with inflammatory arthritis over the course of years, doctors have found that the most important matter is to identify and control the inflammation quickly. And the process for controlling inflammation is similar for most types of inflammatory arthritis, regardless of your specific diagnosis. For example, your doctor might try an anti-inflammatory drug such as ibuprofen, naproxen, celecoxib, rofecoxib or others, or even low-dose glucocorticoids over a period of one to two months, even when an exact diagnosis has not been established.

You may feel a lot better, have less pain and function more easily — all to your benefit. The evidence suggests that as long as your joint inflammation is controlled, there is a low likelihood that you will develop joint damage.

removal of the spleen is required to manage Felty's syndrome effectively.

Connective Tissue Diseases

A number of related diseases, referred to as connective tissue diseases, may be associated with arthritis, and can give the appearance of rheumatoid arthritis. Some of the more common forms of connective tissue disease are described below.

SYSTEMIC LUPUS ERYTHEMATOSUS (LUPUS)

Like rheumatoid arthritis, systemic lupus erythematosus (also called SLE or lupus) is characterized by musculoskeletal pain that is caused by inflammation and an autoimmune response. Almost all people with lupus will test positive for antinuclear antibodies (ANA), but up to one half of those with rheumatoid arthritis also have a positive ANA test.

Arthritis and skin rashes are common in people with lupus. In addition, involvement of vital organs such as the kidney or brain may occur in lupus, leading to serious complications.

SCLERODERMA (SYSTEMIC SCLEROSIS)

This disease is characterized by tightening of the skin. People with scleroderma may experience a discoloration of the hands when exposed to cold (known as Raynaud's phenomenon). This may also be seen in people with rheumatoid arthritis. People with scleroderma may also have involvement of internal organs, in particular the lungs, kidneys and gastrointestinal tract.

Personally Speaking Stories from real people with rheumatoid arthritis

"In the very early stages of my diagnosis with rheumatoid arthritis, my body and mind had become unfamiliar to me. The many daily tasks that had been so routine had all taken on new dimensions. The simple things had become such a chore, and I struggled to accomplish even the smallest of tasks, such as getting dressed and personal hygiene.

The Only Person Who Could Help Was Me
by Cheryl Licastri, Liverpool, NY

"I soon learned that without managing my energies, my efforts had become burdens. The face that I saw wrenching in the mirror with pain was not the person that I had wanted to be. The face was a stranger to me, and one that I had not wanted to know. I knew that the only person who could change that face into one that was more reflective of me, *was me.*

"It was then that my arthritis had become a gift. My life had been awakened, as I stepped out from behind the gray shadows of this disease, and breathed."

POLYMYOSITIS AND DERMATOMYOSITIS

Polymyositis is a disease in which inflammation occurs primarily in muscles. This inflammation can lead to muscle weakness and permanent muscle damage with irreversible weakness.

Some people with polymyositis also develop rashes on their hands, face or trunk, a condition referred to as dermato ("skin") myositis.

VASCULITIS

Vasculitis is an inflammation of the blood vessels that may affect any organ of the body. Some people with vasculitis may have arthritis that is difficult to distinguish from rheumatoid arthritis. To further complicate things, people with rheumatoid arthritis occasionally develop a vasculitis (rheumatoid vasculitis), and it may be difficult to determine which one is the primary condition.

Chapter 6

More Than Joints:

When Other Body Parts Are Affected

Although rheumatoid arthritis most commonly affects your joints, other parts of the body may become involved as well. As we mentioned in Chapter 2, rheumatoid arthritis is called a *systemic* disease, meaning it involves the whole body. The swelling and pain in the joints and other parts of the body result from inflammation. In addition, the process of inflammation is a major reason you are likely to have an overall poor sense of well-being, with fatigue, fevers or weight loss during the course of the disease.

It might be expected that some people with rheumatoid arthritis would have other body organs, in addition to the joints, that are affected by the disease process. When examined carefully, many people with rheumatoid arthritis show some signs of organ involvement. Fortunately, such involvement is generally not severe, and doesn't produce any clinical symptoms. Sometimes, there can be important problems. These are reviewed in this chapter.

The organs most likely to be affected by rheumatoid arthritis include the skin, eyes, mouth, lungs, heart, kidneys, blood cells and spleen. The effects are described in this chapter. Keep in mind, however, that involvement of these organs is not commonly seen in most people with rheumatoid arthritis.

When other organs are affected in people with rheumatoid arthritis, an important consideration is whether the involvement is due to the disease itself, to side effects of the drugs used to treat rheumatoid arthritis, or to both (see box, page 38).

Skin

Rheumatoid nodules are seen at some point in the disease in about one half of people with rheumatoid arthritis. These nodules are actually lumps of tissue that form under the skin, often over bony areas exposed to pressure (such as on the fingers or around the elbow). No treatment is usually necessary, unless the nodule is located in a sensitive spot, such as where a person holds a pencil. The nodules sometimes disappear on their own or with treatment. Interestingly, almost all people who develop these nodules also have rheumatoid factor, although doctors are unsure what (if any) the connection may be.

The drugs used to treat rheumatoid arthritis can also cause problems with the skin. For example, rashes can occur as a side effect of some medications used in rheumatoid arthritis. Blue or purplish bruises sometimes appear on the skin as a result of glucocorticoid use.

The skin is occasionally affected by *vasculitis* (inflammation of the blood vessels), which can cause red dots to appear on the skin. This is a relatively unusual complication, but it may be a clue that the same process is occurring in internal organs such as the lungs or kidneys. Such involvement can have serious consequences if not brought under control, although aggressive treatment with glucocorticoids, methotrexate and other *cytotoxic* drugs (chemicals that destroy cells or prevent their multiplication) usually resolves the problem.

Eyes

There are two important ways in which rheumatoid arthritis might involve the eyes. One, dry eyes, is a component of Sjögren's syndrome (also known as sicca syndrome), which was mentioned in Chapter 5. The problem of dry eyes may be treated by the use of "artificial tears" eye drops. In severe cases, a special surgical procedure may help lubricate the eyes.

To Treat Aggressively or To Back Off – That's the Question

The drugs used to treat rheumatoid arthritis, which are explored in depth in Chapter 11, are powerful. That is one reason doctors carefully monitor their patients for possible side effects. However, one problem in rheumatoid arthritis is to determine whether the complication is an effect of the disease process, in which the body's own immune system seemingly turns against itself, or if a drug is causing the problem.

This is where the dilemma occurs: When possible side effects are noted, the tendency is to back off from aggressive treatment by reducing dosages or stopping drugs altogether. However, in some people this approach may be a mistake.

If you face a similar situation, talk to your doctor about the options available. It should always be a consideration that organ involvement in some (but certainly not all) people with rheumatoid arthritis may more likely be a component of the disease than a side effect of treatment. The disease should continue to be treated aggressively – that is, with strong doses of powerful drugs.

Another condition that may be associated with rheumatoid arthritis is an inflammation of the eyes, known as *scleritis*. This condition may require treatment with eye drops, as well as aggressive anti-inflammatory medications. A rare complication of scleritis is *scleromalacia perforans*, in which the eye can be permanently damaged by severe inflammation. People with rheumatoid arthritis who develop redness of their eyes that persists longer than a few days should be examined by an eye-care professional to determine if treatment for scleritis is needed. However, it is again emphasized that severe eye inflammation is rare.

Mouth

In addition to the eyes, the mouth may become dry in Sjögren's syndrome, because of a decrease in the body's production of saliva. People with this syndrome should drink plenty of fluids to keep the mouth

---

Personally Speaking Stories from real people with rheumatoid arthritis

"**B**eep, beep, beep…my alarm sounds at 6:06 a.m. each day. I react by turning over and looking at the clock wondering what happened to the night. I leave the house at around 7 a.m., only after I have taken 10 pills and eaten breakfast to help the pills work. When I get to my locker at school, my locker partner opens it for me, because my hands just don't want to work at that hour.

High School, Homework and Arthritis
by Carly Snyder, Mentor, OH

"In the evenings, after homework and dinner, I take five more pills and go up to my room, hoping my mom will forget my shot. She never does. As soon as I hear her coming up the stairs, I start to tear up. I smell the rubbing alcohol that I must put on my thigh, and I almost throw up. I pinch my skin and shove the shot into my leg. It stings and I feel the liquid spread throughout my body.

"Extracurricular activities keep me busy. Instead of running, I plan assemblies and dances. Instead of anticipating a soccer game, I look forward to a trip with the law club to Toronto. I teach astronomy to elementary school students, swim for diabetes, walk for MS, teach Sunday school at church, and collect toys for tots. As a result of all my hard work, this year I was tapped for membership in National Honor Society.

"When I tell people at school about my arthritis, I think it scares them. So I always try to make a funny comment such as, 'I'm a 60-year-old trapped in a 17-year-old's body!' When they see that I can deal with it and laugh about it, it eases their minds. I truly believe the best medicine can't, and will never be, prescribed for anyone, because laughter is found within and around everyone."

moist, especially when eating dry foods. Good dental hygiene is a must, as bacteria tend to flourish without the usual flow of saliva in the mouth.

Mouth sores or oral ulcers are a frequent complication of treatment with methotrexate, and sometimes with injectable gold. This problem can often be controlled by using mouthwashes and by reducing the dose of methotrexate.

Lungs

Involvement of the lungs is not uncommon in people with rheumatoid arthritis. Inflammation of the lining of the lungs, known as *pleurisy*, can cause pain when taking a deep breath. In general, the inflammation will subside with standard anti-inflammatory treatments for rheumatoid arthritis.

Occasionally, people with rheumatoid arthritis may develop scarring, called *pulmonary fibrosis,* that leads to progressive shortness of breath.

Medications used to treat rheumatoid arthritis, such as methotrexate, can sometimes affect the lungs, a complication known as "methotrexate lung" or "methotrexate pneumonia." The pneumonia generally goes away when the methotrexate is stopped. Most people can safely resume taking methotrexate a few weeks after an episode of methotrexate pneumonia.

Similar drug-induced pneumonias have also been reported with other drugs used in rheumatoid arthritis, including injectable gold and penicillamine.

Sometimes it is difficult to tell whether a lung problem results from rheumatoid arthritis or from a drug. In such cases, you and your doctor must decide how to handle the situation, or you may consider other diagnostic testing. This is another example of how the condition and its treatments must be monitored over time.

Heart

In most people, the heart itself is not directly affected by rheumatoid arthritis. On occasion, however, people with rheumatoid arthritis may develop *pericarditis* (inflammation of the lining surrounding the heart), leading to chest pain or discomfort and requiring direct treatment.

Kidneys

The kidneys' function is to remove waste products from the body. In some people with rheumatoid arthritis, kidney function (as measured by the blood urea nitrogen [BUN] or creatinine) may be reduced. Problems with kidney function in people with rheumatoid arthritis are more likely to be related to side effects of the drugs used to treat rheumatoid arthritis – such as cyclosporine (*Neoral*) or a nonsteroidal anti-inflammatory drug (NSAID) – than to the disease itself. If you are taking one of these drugs, your doctor will monitor your renal (kidney) function at periodic intervals.

Blood-Forming Cells

People with rheumatoid arthritis may have *anemia* (reduction in the number of red blood cells) that is sometimes called the anemia of chronic disease. No special treatment is necessary for this condition, which improves as the level of inflammation in the body is brought under control.

Occasionally, people with rheumatoid arthritis may develop other types of anemias. *Iron-deficiency anemia* usually results from the loss of blood in the intestinal tract, for example from an ulcer or polyp, or in women, from blood loss in menstrual periods. Iron-replacement treatment can correct this problem. *Pernicious anemia* (due to a lack of vitamin B-12) is now relatively rare; when it does occur it can be corrected with vitamin B-12 injections and/or folic acid. A decrease in the number of white blood cells is seen in Felty's syndrome (see Chapter 5), which is associated with enlargement of the spleen.

People with very active inflammation may have high levels of blood platelets. These levels return toward normal when the inflammation is controlled. Aggressive drug treatment of rheumatoid arthritis may result in decreased numbers of platelets (called *thrombocytopenia*) if the bone marrow is suppressed, emphasizing the need for periodic monitoring.

Similarly, the use of certain medications may lead to decreased numbers of white blood cells in the body, which is another reason that periodic monitoring and blood counts are necessary.

Spleen

Felty's syndrome is the name given to a condition that occurs when people with rheumatoid arthritis have a reduced number of white blood cells and an enlarged spleen. Some doctors consider this syndrome to be linked to a more severe form of rheumatoid arthritis. In general, the treatment for this condition should be aggressive, as in severe rheumatoid arthritis. Of note, there appears to be an increased risk of non-Hodgkin's lymphoma in people with rheumatoid arthritis who develop Felty's syndrome.

Chapter 7

The Long Haul:

What To Expect Over Time

Anyone who has a chronic disease is often almost as concerned about what will happen over the long haul as what is happening today. This is completely understandable, especially when the chronic disease is rheumatoid arthritis. As chronic diseases go, rheumatoid arthritis is particularly frustrating: there may be periods of flare and periods of seeming remission, times when your joints are stiff and painful and times when you feel fine. It may be difficult to know what to expect on a day-to-day basis.

People's expectations are often greatly influenced by their own experiences in life. Perhaps you may know someone who had rheumatoid arthritis that was quite severe, so that she had to quit working or was unable to take care of herself. You might be intensely worried about experiencing such an outcome. On the other hand, you might know someone with a very mild case of rheumatoid arthritis, and you may think it unlikely that you will have any significant problems coping with the disease yourself.

In this chapter we will talk about some of the things that may happen over time if you have rheumatoid arthritis. Because all people with rheumatoid arthritis are individuals, it is practically impossible to predict exactly how anyone's disease will progress over time. Even so, there are some general guidelines that can help you and your doctor establish a reasonable possibility of what might happen over the course of this chronic disease.

Making a Prediction – Some General Guidelines

Some clues that can help determine the long-term course and severity of rheumatoid arthritis – such as the number of joints that are involved or the level of C-reactive protein (CRP) in the blood – cannot be influenced by you. There are other clues that you *can* affect, however, such as how quickly treatment is started and how well you can adapt to the challenges of dealing with rheumatoid arthritis. These general guidelines about your long-term outcome include the following:

• **The actual rate of progression of the disease.** This progression is what some people call the "natural history" or the course that the disease takes in your body. Careful monitoring over several months is often the most helpful method to predict the course of disease. A combination of factors may determine the rate of progression, including the level of pain, fatigue, tenderness and swelling; level of function and disability; and the number of involved joints. Lab tests may provide more information.

• **How quickly treatment is begun.** For some people, there can be a long interval between the first signs of rheumatoid arthritis and when the disease is diagnosed and treatment is started. This means that the inflammation in the body is not controlled. It becomes chronic and leads to the beginning of long-term damage to the joints.

• **How aggressively the disease is treated.** It has become very clear in recent years that treatment for rheumatoid arthritis should be aggressive. That is, medications should be strong enough to bring the inflammation under control, not just to reduce the symptoms, as early as possible. Reducing symptoms may reduce the underlying damage being caused to the joints, but long-term damage to joints can still occur.

• **How the individual is coping with the disease.** It has been shown that people who

feel they are "in control" of their chronic disease tend to have a better long-term outlook. This type of coping is often referred to as *self-efficacy*, and it is an important cornerstone of this book. Other components of effective coping include using joint-preserving techniques, exercising and keeping a positive outlook.

Another Clue: Your Disease Type

One important source of confusion when it comes to predicting the future of your disease course is that some people who meet the criteria for rheumatoid arthritis (discussed in Chapter 3) will actually turn out to have a disease course that goes away on its own over a few months. Others turn out to have a disease course with inflammation and joint involvement that seems to get worse over time (especially if not treated). Still others seem to travel a middle road, their disease well controlled by anti-inflammatory medications (see box, page 45).

TYPE I DISEASE

In the late 1960s, large studies involving the entire population of certain areas were conducted to see how many people might meet the criteria for rheumatoid arthritis. As it turned out, about two percent of the population met these criteria. About 75 percent of those who met the criteria did not show evidence of having rheumatoid arthritis three to five years later. Among those who initially met the criteria for rheumatoid arthritis but did not have evidence of having the disease after five years, apparently many never saw a doctor about their symptoms.

The Three Types of Rheumatoid Arthritis

	TYPE I	TYPE II	TYPE III
Progression	Spontaneous remission	Minimal disease progress	Serious disease progress
Percentage of people with type	5-20%	5-20%	60-90%
How is it distinguished?	Negative Rheumatoid Factor	Lasts more than six months, positive lab findings	Lasts more than six months, positive lab findings
Also called	Inflammatory arthritis, reactive arthritis, post-viral arthritis	Mild rheumatoid arthritis	Persistent inflammatory symmetrical arthritis

It now seems likely that if a person has symptoms that meet the criteria for rheumatoid arthritis for less than six months, there is a good chance that the condition will go away on its own. As doctors have learned more about this early stage of disease, they often recognize this type of arthritis that does not tend to progress. In fact, they may call it something other than rheumatoid arthritis – perhaps "reactive arthritis" or "inflammatory polyarthritis." The term rheumatoid arthritis is now usually reserved for a more severe disease process. The type of arthritis that goes away within six months has been called "Type I disease."

TYPE II DISEASE

Most people who meet the criteria for rheumatoid arthritis and have experienced arthritis in symmetrical joints – that is, both wrists, both hands and so on – for longer than six months do not experience a spontaneous remission of their symptoms. A minority of these people with progressive rheumatoid arthritis, from five percent to 20 percent, may have a mild disease course that can be controlled with less aggressive therapy, such as with nonsteroidal anti-inflammatory drugs (NSAIDs) alone. This form of rheumatoid arthritis is referred to as "Type II disease." Although Type II disease is progressive, it tends to cause less severe damage to joints and often does not affect other parts of the body.

TYPE III DISEASE

Most people who have symptoms of rheumatoid arthritis for longer than six months will have what is known as "persistent inflammatory symmetrical arthritis" (PISA) or "Type III disease." This is the most severe type of the disease, affecting 60 percent to 90 percent of people who have rheumatoid arthritis that is monitored in clinicians' offices. The symptoms usually cannot be controlled with NSAIDs alone; stronger disease-modifying antirheumatic drugs (known as DMARDs, see Chapter 11) are needed as well to control inflammation and prevent damage.

Progressive or Type III rheumatoid arthritis has traditionally been recognized as having severe long-term consequences. However, these consequences should be put in perspective at this time. New information, new drugs and more aggressive treatment strategies have combined to greatly improve the long-term outlook for people with Type III rheumatoid arthritis. Because of these advances, doctors are hopeful that the sort of joint damage that was common 20 years ago will now be considered a thing of the past.

Why It's Important To See a Doctor

As you can see, during the first six months that you have symptoms of rheumatoid arthritis, the disease may go away on its own. Why, then, is it important to see a doctor as quickly as possible if you think you may have rheumatoid arthritis?

First, it is worthwhile to see a doctor just to make sure that what you have *is* rheumatoid arthritis. As mentioned in Chapter 4, a number of diseases can mimic rheumatoid arthritis – some of which have very different treatments and outcomes. An experienced doctor will consider all the evidence and make a diagnosis.

Second, it is wise to establish some benchmark measurements during the early months of the disease. This will provide important information to your doctor as he or she monitors the progression of disease over time. In these early months, the doctor will look for persistent joint swelling, rheumatoid factor and even early evidence of changes on X-rays.

Third, if there is evidence of progressive disease at an early visit, it becomes possible to begin treatment to control inflammation – thus helping to prevent damage to joints down the line. Until recently, many people, including doctors and people with rheumatoid arthritis, often felt that the treatment was worse than the disease. However, new and effective drugs, with fewer side effects, have changed the situation dramatically. Early treatment with these drugs has been shown to have a big impact on the long-term outlook for people with rheumatoid arthritis.

Finally, there is nothing wrong with seeing your doctor about a condition that may get better on its own. In fact, about one half of all visits to physicians involve such situations. In this case, it truly is better to be safe than sorry.

What Changes You Can Expect

During the 1980s, several rheumatology centers reported information that surprised health professionals: Many people with rheumatoid arthritis experienced much poorer than predicted long-term outcomes. At that time, most doctors believed that the outcomes of most people with rheumatoid arthritis were relatively favorable over the long term, with only a few patients experiencing poor outcomes. The reports suggested that most people with rheumatoid arthritis were experiencing extensive joint damage seen in the progression of their X-rays, severe declines in ability to function, frequent work disability, and even shortened life span.

Those observations led to renewed efforts to improve long-term outcomes, and the care of people with rheumatoid arthritis has changed dramatically, particularly over the last decade. Indeed, there is much evidence that in the 1990s, people who had regular care by a rheumatologist and who received more aggressive therapy, including new and more effective drugs, had much better outcomes than in earlier periods. In order to better understand why these changes in the treatment of rheumatoid arthritis were needed, let's review some of the changes that are seen in individuals with this chronic disease.

X-RAY CHANGES

Over time, X-rays show joint damage in almost all people with rheumatoid arthritis who are untreated or who are not receiving aggressive treatment to control the disease. In fact, about seven of 10 people who have

Personally Speaking   Stories from real people with rheumatoid arthritis

"**H**aving suffered with rheumatoid arthritis for more than 20 years, I've tried almost every NSAID and so-called newly discovered miracle drug, from gold shots to *Celebrex* and *Vioxx*, mostly to short-lived relief. Prednisone has brought 'instant relief,' but it's entirely too dangerous to continue taking it for too extended a stretch, and very difficult to reduce to a small dosage.

What Helps Me Get Through the Day
by Betty McKelvey, Beaufort, MO

"I read avidly about each new drug discovery. I know I will *not* be financially able to try these new drugs sold at inflated prices at the pharmacy.

"In 1998, the YMCA opened a small facility with a wonderfully heated pool. The aquatics program by the Y, in conjunction with the Arthritis Foundation Eastern Missouri chapter, has changed my life. Being in warm water, up to my shoulders, gently exercising each joint from my neck down to my toes, gives me more relief than any high-priced medication. The educational pointers about arthritis, along with happy group participation, is what I look forward to each day."

rheumatoid arthritis develop joint changes that can be seen on X-rays within two years. A magnetic resonance imaging (MRI) scan may show damage to joints even earlier.

Although damage to joints can be improved with medication, most joint damage is not reversible. In most people, the most rapid damage occurs early in the disease process, when inflammation is present. This is yet another reason disease-modifying antirheumatic drugs or combinations of drugs should be used, as it is crucial to stop joint damage early.

CHANGES IN FUNCTION

Another way to measure the progress of rheumatoid arthritis is to observe an individual's ability to perform usual activities such as dressing, bathing, walking and running errands. Overall, more than 90 percent of people with rheumatoid arthritis report having some problems in doing their usual activities, and losses in function appear to occur most rapidly during the first few years of the disease.

Under traditional medical care in the 1980s, the majority of people with rheumatoid arthritis experienced greater difficulty completing their daily activities over a five-year period. Now that treatment is more aggressive, health-care professionals have a new understanding of the biopsychosocial approach to treatment (see Chapter 1) and people with rheumatoid arthritis are more involved in managing their arthritis, these numbers have begun to improve.

It is important to prevent losses of function by treating with drugs and other therapies. But if functional losses occur, how can they be handled? Family members may help complete some additional chores around the house. Special aids and devices can be purchased to help with specific tasks such as cooking or dressing. Also, a little advance planning can help you to pace yourself. Ideas like these will be discussed in greater detail in the next section of this book.

WORK DISABILITY

One of the more serious consequences of rheumatoid arthritis is work disability. In fact, some figures show that more than 50 percent of people with rheumatoid arthritis become unable to work after 10 years. This translates into almost one million people in the United States alone who may experience work disability because of this disease.

Interestingly, the severity of disease does not accurately predict who will become disabled from work. There are complex factors that determine whether a person becomes unable to work, including the person's age, occupation and the amount of control the person has over the pace of his or her job.

A number of resources are available to help people with disabilities continue to work (see p. 49). Since the passage of the Americans with Disabilities Act (ADA) in 1990, most employers are required by law to provide reasonable accommodations to help their employees keep working. For example, if you must stand all day to supervise employees, you are within your rights to discuss job modifications with your employer.

You may be concerned about whether to continue working. Perhaps friends, relatives or even some doctors may be insisting that you give up your job. But remember that this choice should be made only after you have explored all the alternatives carefully, both with your doctor and with your employer. Many job modifications cost little and can allow you to keep working without exhausting yourself or putting pressure on your joints. People who continue to work outside the home may have better long-term outcomes, although this may reflect in large part their better clinical status.

LIFE SPAN

Several conditions such as infection, pulmonary disease, renal disease or gastrointestinal problems are more common in people with rheumatoid arthritis. In

If You Are Facing Work Disability

There are many resources available to people with rheumatoid arthritis who may be facing work disability. Career counseling and vocational testing services of the state-federal vocational rehabilitation program are available at no cost and are located in all 50 states. These and some other resources are listed below.

GOVERNMENT-SPONSORED VOCATIONAL REHABILITATION SERVICES

Most people with rheumatoid arthritis should be eligible for the following services: vocational counseling and testing; job placement; assistance with resume preparation and interview skills; payment for job accommodations, training, education and travel.

INDEPENDENT LIVING CENTERS

These centers provide advocacy services and programs that enable people with disabilities to live on their own.

JOB ACCOMMODATION NETWORK

This free consulting service, operated by the President's Committee on Employment of People with Disabilities, provides information about the Americans with Disabilities Act and types of job accommodations. (800) 526-7234.

DISABILITY AND BUSINESS TECHNICAL ASSISTANCE CENTERS

Centers are available in each region of the country to advise businesses and individuals about accommodations. (800) 949-4232.

THE ARTHRITIS FOUNDATION

This organization has excellent brochures on dealing with employment challenges experienced by people with arthritis. (800) 283-7800.

addition, studies have shown that having severe rheumatoid arthritis may decrease an individual's life span by as much as 10 to 15 years compared to someone without the disease. Many factors are involved in determining how the disease affects survival, including age, number of involved joints and ability to carry out daily activities.

On a positive note, new and more effective medications and treatments (which will be discussed fully in Chapter 11) are likely to reduce these serious complications and enhance the life span of patients with rheumatoid arthritis. This underscores the importance of early, aggressive treatment of rheumatoid arthritis.

Part Two

Medical Management:
What to Expect

Chapter 8

Keeping Tabs:

Evaluating and Monitoring Your Rheumatoid Arthritis

We have already discussed some of the difficulties of making a diagnosis of rheumatoid arthritis. Because this is a chronic disease, it is equally important to evaluate disease activity over time and to monitor the effectiveness of treatment to prevent long-term damage.

Experts have spent much time and effort figuring out ways to measure rheumatoid arthritis disease activity in individuals, so the best treatment plan for each person can be determined. Even though the disease course varies from person to person, there are certain guidelines or indicators that can be used to help doctors find out how well the current treatment is working, or whether an additional or alternative drug is needed.

Some of the same tests or measures that may be used initially to diagnose rheumatoid arthritis may also be used to evaluate and monitor its course. For example, an examination of the joints by a doctor quickly reveals information about joint swelling, tenderness and range of motion, including how many joints are involved. In addition, X-rays, laboratory tests, functional measures and patient questionnaires all provide valuable information when used appropriately at regular intervals. By asking for input directly from the person with arthritis, patient questionnaires are an especially rich source of

information on functional capacity, pain, fatigue, psychological distress and other consequences of rheumatoid arthritis.

In this chapter, we will discuss some of the methods and measures used to evaluate disease activity, as well as to monitor for drug effectiveness and possibly for adverse effects.

Although there are many different ways to evaluate and monitor rheumatoid arthritis, it is possible to group these measures into three fairly broad categories.

- **Measures of inflammatory activity.** These measures are generally most useful in the first few years of rheumatoid arthritis, when severe inflammation is usually present without any damage. Useful measures of inflammation include joint tenderness and swelling, as well as laboratory tests such as sedimentation rate and C-reactive protein. These measures can change over time to show whether a drug is effective in reducing inflammation.

• **Measures of damage.** Long-term joint damage is one of the more worrisome aspects of rheumatoid arthritis disease activity. Measures used to assess joint damage include exams of mobility and joint alignment, X-rays, or specialized tests of function such as walk times or button tests. These measures are used to evaluate quality of life, because joint damage in part determines a person's ability to carry out daily activities. Measures of damage mostly assess changes over months to years.

• **Measures of outcome.** Outcomes are the consequences of disease that are of most interest to a person with arthritis. They include loss of function, work disability, joint destruction and costs associated with the disease. Outcomes may be followed in long-term studies (studies that follow a group of individuals over the course of many years), or may be evaluated by sifting through information such as applications for disability related to rheumatoid arthritis.

One thing to keep in mind is that these three types of measures do not necessarily measure the same thing. For example, joint tenderness is a very effective measure of dis-

ease activity, but it is not meaningfully associated with changes that show up on X-rays. Although this may be hard to understand, it is important. Serious concerns have emerged over the last decade as evidence has shown, in some cases, that measures of inflammatory activity may be stable – but damage to the joints and/or organs still may progress. This problem emerged as people were treated under a more cautious, less aggressive approach. These findings suggest that partial control of inflammation may not prevent long-term damage, which is one reason doctors now try to control the inflammation as strongly and as quickly as possible in rheumatoid arthritis.

Joint Examinations

Because rheumatoid arthritis involves the joints, a joint examination is one of the key features used to evaluate disease activity. Changes in your joint count, or the number of joints that are tender or swollen, are a measure of the inflammation associated with rheumatoid arthritis. Joint counts provide a way for doctors to note disease progression or improvement. In addition, your doctor will probably look for any pain during motion, limitation in the motion of your joint or joint malalignment. When the structures in the joint fail to align properly, joint function is hampered.

There are several different methods used for joint counts, ranging from the simple (a rating of normal or abnormal for each joint) to the complex (four or more possible gradations for each joint). In general, the simpler measures have been found to perform just as well as the more complex ones. The number of joints counted also varies, from as few as 28 to as many as 70. In long-term studies, joint counts have proved useful in assessing, monitoring and even predicting the course of rheumatoid arthritis in individuals.

X-rays and Other Imaging Techniques

X-rays (also called *radiographs*) are useful for showing specific types of changes associated with rheumatoid arthritis. Disease evidence provided by these measures include narrowing of the joint space, erosion of the structures in the joint and malalignment of the joint.

In addition, X-rays can show changes of osteoporosis, which is associated with rheumatoid arthritis itself as well as with some drugs used to treat rheumatoid arthritis.

X-rays are useful for evaluating joint damage. Sometimes your doctor will take what are known as "baseline X-rays" when you are first diagnosed with rheumatoid arthritis.

Personally Speaking Stories from real people with rheumatoid arthritis

"I've always been one of those people who sees the glass as half-full. My optimism was put to the test 14 years ago, when I was diagnosed with rheumatoid arthritis. One day, I was a healthy, energetic woman. The next day, I walked with a cane.

Optimism Rewarded: Hooked on Fitness and Nutrition
by Katherina Chrysostomou Colston, Adairsville, GA

Nothing had prepared me for this change. The world as I knew it had come to an end. From then on, I never knew what to expect – if I would make it to work or to my daughter's school play. Simple things like washing my hair and getting dressed became Herculean tasks.

"Five years ago, my life changed again. I became hooked on fitness and proper nutrition. It started by subscribing to *Arthritis Today* magazine. I began learning more about my illness and how to cope with it. As my body became stronger, my spirit began to soar. I became courageous, enrolling in and graduating from the Atlanta School of Fitness and Nutrition. Last summer, my daughter and I power-walked the 10-K Peachtree Road Race.

"Although winters are not kind to people with arthritis, I still exercise daily to keep my joints, muscles and connective tissue strong. My goal is to inspire others. That's why I'm studying for my certification as a fitness trainer. My message is that people with arthritis can do just about anything. It just takes patience and courage."

These X-rays are used as a basis for comparison through the years so that any changes are readily noted.

Some of the newer imaging techniques that have been developed – such as magnetic resonance imaging (MRI) and ultrasound scanning – enable doctors to find evidence of inflammation before joint damage occurs. X-rays are less sensitive and primarily assess damaged joints. These newer measures may be used more often in the future for evaluating and monitoring disease activity.

Laboratory Tests

The two most widely used laboratory tests to assess inflammation are the erythrocyte sedimentation rate (ESR or sed rate), and C-reactive protein (CRP). As we noted before, these tests are not always abnormal in people with rheumatoid arthritis – only 60 percent to 70 percent of people with the disease show elevated levels of these measures. However, in people who do have elevated levels, the ESR and CRP can provide valuable information about disease activity over time.

Blood counts often are used to monitor for adverse effects that can occur from medications used to treat rheumatoid arthritis, such as methotrexate. These tests may be repeated periodically. For example, a low white blood cell count can indicate suppression of blood cell formation in the bone marrow. Low red blood cell counts suggest anemia, and can be caused by small amounts of bleeding in the gastrointestinal tract when taking certain drugs such as non-steroidal anti-inflammatories.

A urinalysis, a test done on a sample of urine to determine its contents, may also be done. The tests show whether urine contains red blood cells, protein or a variety of other abnormal substances. Again, these measures are used to monitor the effects of strong medications.

Liver function tests measure the levels of enzymes produced by the liver. The level may be elevated in people taking certain drugs for rheumatoid arthritis, including methotrexate and leflunomide (*Arava*). The tests are usually repeated every four to eight weeks for individuals using these drugs, and the results are closely monitored.

Physical Function Measures

Physical measures of function may indicate both inflammatory activity and evidence of long-term joint damage. These measures (discussed in Chapter 3) may be repeated for comparison from one visit to another. Some of the more commonly used measures include grip strength, walking time and manual dexterity (button test and others).

Self-Report Questionnaires

Self-report questionnaires provide a way to measure symptoms and concerns that are difficult to quantify by other medical methods such as laboratory tests or X-rays. They may ask questions about pain, fatigue, loss in functional status and psychological distress. Improvements or worsening in these areas have been shown to be documented best by patients' self-report measures. As with other evaluative measures, they are usually repeated at regular intervals. The most commonly used measures are described in Chapter 3.

Patient questionnaires provide another avenue for your input, by asking for information that only you can provide. Many doctors feel that these self-report measures are the most effective way to monitor individual changes in status over five to 10 years. By taking the time to fill out these questionnaires as completely, accurately and honestly as possible, you can work with your doctor and other health-care professionals to develop the best treatment plan and help evaluate its effectiveness over time.

Chapter 9

Your Medical Managers:

Getting To Know the Players

Now we have explored what rheumatoid arthritis is and how it can affect your body. Let's delve into some of the keys to the medical management of rheumatoid arthritis: What does it involve and how can you participate?

For the most part, people think of "medical management" in terms of drugs or medications prescribed by a doctor. It's true that doctors and drugs are cornerstones of treatment. In a chronic disease like rheumatoid arthritis, however, there are many more actions that you and your health-care professionals can take to help manage the effects of the disease.

In this chapter, we discuss the health professionals with whom you may interact. In the next chapter, we will discuss self-management. Then we will review the various drugs you may take for rheumatoid arthritis.

Who Are Your Medical Managers?

You may already have gotten the idea that you and your doctor should form a partnership in managing your arthritis. But what is meant by the term "medical managers," and what other health professionals are involved?

Your medical management or health-care team may include anyone that might assist you in receiving comprehensive care for *your* rheumatoid arthritis. Like the disease itself, your individual needs may vary when it comes to your medical managers. Some people do well working with only their doctor and his or her office staff (including nurses or nurse practitioners), others turn to one or two health professionals or therapists, whereas others will need the resources of a larger number of professionals involved in their care.

To use an old metaphor, think of your arthritis care in terms of a play to be staged. The play should not be a "one man show," nor should it be a cast of thousands. Instead, envision it as an ensemble production, in which each player has a very particular and necessary role. In some acts, only two or three players will appear; in others, the whole cast may be on stage. Finally, you need to view yourself as not only playing a key part, but being the director as well. It will be up to you to decide which players can be used most effectively in which scenes.

Meeting the Players

Many different specialists, therapists and other health professionals may be involved in the management of your condition, depending on the problems or symptoms you encounter, and the availability of services in your area. The following is a list and brief description of some of the health-care professionals who may play a role in your treatment.

DOCTORS

Family physicians, *general practitioners* and *primary care physicians* provide medical care for adults and children with different types of arthritis and related conditions. These doctors provide the cornerstone of medical treatment for your general health, and manage common additional medical problems such as high blood pressure or gastrointestinal distress. These general doctors can also help you locate a specialist. Every person should have a family physician or internist as a primary care doctor – a specialist should not be your only doctor.

Internists specialize in internal medicine and treating adult diseases. They may be general internists who act as primary care physicians, or they may be subspecialists

who have completed additional training in specific types of disease. A general internist provides general care to adults and often helps select subspecialists. Internists should not be confused with *interns*, who are doctors doing a year's training in a hospital after graduating from medical school.

Rheumatologists are internists who have further training to treat people with arthritis or related diseases that affect the joints, muscles, bones, skin and other tissues. Most people with rheumatoid arthritis are referred to a rheumatologist at least at some point in their care for special assessment and treatment. Some rheumatologists may also have training in pediatrics, orthopaedics, physical medicine, sports medicine or other medical fields.

Orthopaedic surgeons or *orthopaedists* are doctors who specialize in diseases of the bone. The general area of care for specialists in orthopaedics involves mechanical problems of bones and joints, in contrast to inflammatory problems such as rheumatoid arthritis. Orthopaedists are the doctors who set fractures, examine or repair a knee or other joint through an arthroscope, or replace a damaged hip, knee or other joint with a metal or plastic joint. Many orthopaedists subspecialize in particular areas, such as hand surgery, sports medicine, joint replacement, etc.

When a person develops musculoskeletal pain, it is often not clear whether the problem is mechanical, inflammatory, or even based on some other type of cause, such as an infection or metabolic problem. Therefore, people with rheumatoid arthritis may be referred at first to an orthopaedic surgeon.

Pediatricians treat childhood diseases. A child who develops arthritis will see a pediatrician at first. Certain pediatricians known as *pediatric rheumatologists* specialize in the care of arthritis in children. These specialist pediatricians are usually located only in large cities or medical centers. A visit to such a specialist can be extremely helpful to a child with juvenile arthritis.

Physiatrists are doctors who direct physical therapy and rehabilitation programs.

Comprehensive rehabilitation programs may have been more common 10 or 20 years ago when joint destruction was seen in most people with rheumatoid arthritis. Inflammation is better controlled today, and this type of treatment may be less necessary than in the past for people with rheumatoid arthritis. However, physical therapy still plays a major role in treatment for some people with rheumatoid arthritis.

Podiatrists or *chiropodists* are doctors with particular training in the care of the feet. These doctors may be extremely helpful to

Personally Speaking Stories from real people with rheumatoid arthritis

"In December 1996, I started experiencing severe pain in my feet. I could be simply blow-drying my hair and notice my feet swelling and turning purple. I just assumed it must be due to my cheerleading, that I was on my feet too much. I became very fatigued, with little strength. My doctor ran X-rays on my feet, checked my lymph nodes, and finally, took some blood tests. This is where I was diagnosed with rheumatoid arthritis. My first thought was that I was only 16 – only old people get this! I was sadly mistaken.

Waiting on My Miracle
by Tiffany Hadden, Eclectic, AL

"All the simple things in my life quickly became challenges. It got to the point where I felt like a baby, and constantly needed someone to assist me. My mom got into the habit of coming upstairs every morning to put clothes on me, tie my shoes, and even fix my hair. Buttoning things and pulling zippers, opening a jug of milk or even pouring it all became hurdles that I couldn't overcome.

"I get really mad at myself. If you comfort me, I get defensive, because I want to do it for myself. Yet if you don't, I feel that I am of no importance. It's a really thin line between the two. Somehow, my family seems to distinguish that line. The morning that it took both of my parents to carry me down the stairs, they acted like it was no big deal. That helped me cope with the situation. Life has become a battle, full of challenges to overcome every day. But I know that I have a miracle with my name on it."

certain people with extensive disease involvement of their feet.

Psychiatrists are medical doctors who treat mental or emotional problems that need special attention. They can prescribe medications for treating the problems. *Psychologists* are also trained to treat mental or emotional problems, but have a doctor of philosophy (PhD) rather than a doctor of medicine degree (MD) and therefore do not prescribe medications. Psychiatrists and psychologists can be very helpful to people who have rheumatoid arthritis, as it is not uncommon that psychological issues affect their daily lives.

OTHER HEALTH PROFESSIONALS

Some *nurses* and *nurse practitioners* are trained in arthritis and related illnesses and can assist your doctor with treatment. They also help teach you about your treatment program and can answer many of your questions or direct you to other resources for information.

Physicians' assistants are trained, certified and licensed to assist physicians by recording medical history and performing the physical examination, diagnosis and treatment of commonly encountered medical problems under the supervision of a licensed physician.

Physical therapists can show you exercises to help keep your muscles strong and your joints from becoming stiff. They can help you learn how to use special equipment to move better. Some physical therapists are trained to design individualized fitness programs for cardiovascular health maintenance and weight control. In general, physical

therapists are concerned with larger joints – shoulders, hips and knees – and broad exercises, in contrast to occupational therapists, who are concerned with the hands and fine motor coordination.

Rehabilitation counselors can work with you to find solutions to work-related problems, such as job retraining or workplace modification.

Occupational therapists can teach you how to reduce strain on your joints while doing everyday activities. They can fit you with splints and other devices, if needed, to help reduce stress on your joints. Their role is mostly for problems with the small joints of the hands, and occasionally with arms and shoulders.

Pharmacists fill your prescriptions for medicines and can explain the actions and side effects of particular drugs. Pharmacists can tell you how different medicines work together and can answer questions about over-the-counter medications.

Social workers can help you access community resources and find solutions to social and financial problems related to your arthritis. They may be of particular help in family situations such as helping to redistribute household responsibilities.

Getting the Most From Your Medical Managers

Communication is the key to getting the most benefit from your health-care professionals. The relationships you develop will probably be long-term ones, and will require work on both parts to develop trust and communication – much like a business partnership or a marriage. You should feel comfortable expressing your fears, asking questions you may think are "stupid," and negotiating a treatment plan that all are satisfied with, without feeling that the health professionals are putting you down or are not interested in your concerns.

There are two things to remember that will help to open (and keep open) the lines of communication. First, try to keep in mind that your doctor or therapist is only human. He or she gets tired, has headaches and even experiences bad days like you do. In addition, it is frustrating not to be able to cure someone with a chronic condition like arthritis. Arthritis health professionals must take their satisfaction from seeing improvements – such as an enhanced quality of life or fewer damaged joints – rather than cures.

Second, remember that the biggest threat to a good relationship and good communication is lack of time. When time is short, there may not be enough time to fully explain things or explore options. Your health professionals' anxiety about time may lead to rushed messages that you misunderstand. Remember – different health professionals can complement each other in some areas. More than one may be able to provide answers to some of your questions.

Taking P.A.R.T.

One way you can maximize the resources of your medical management team is by using a method called "Taking P.A.R.T."

This involves preparing a list of questions or concerns before your visit, asking questions, repeating what you heard and taking action by participating as fully as you can in treatment and management decisions.

Preparing can involve making and keeping your appointment, keeping a diary or journal of your symptoms and your medications, and writing down the questions you want answered. If you don't want to make a list of all your medications, including dosages, bring all your medicine bottles with you. It's all too easy to forget about important questions or exact dosages of drugs in the hustle and bustle of the doctor's office.

Asking your questions may take a little time, but your doctor or health-care professional understands these are valid concerns you have about your disease or your treatment. Bringing a prioritized list of questions to your appointment can save time and may bring up valuable information concerning your treatment.

Repeating the information or instructions you receive back to your health-care profes-

Take P.A.R.T.

To get the most out of your contacts with your medical management team, remember to take P.A.R.T.:

Prepare a list of questions, concerns and symptoms.

Ask questions.

Repeat what you have heard.

Take action to reduce barriers to treatments.

sional ensures that you heard the information correctly and that you understand it. Ask for any available written handouts or instructions. Taking notes may also help you remember complicated instructions.

Taking action by participating in decisions about treatment is especially important because this allows you to share information about your goals and preferences. Let your doctor or other health professional know about your feelings, your lifestyle and your concerns. If something does not work, let him or her know so you can try something else.

Chapter 10

Medical Management:

Effective Strategies for Treatment

In this book we want to emphasize to you that good living with rheumatoid arthritis involves much more than drugs. Self-management, exercise and a positive outlook can make a big difference in how you feel on a day-to-day basis. Nonetheless, we must remember that almost no one can live as well as possible with rheumatoid arthritis without drug treatment. Although there is no cure, excellent control of inflammation to reduce pain and functional limitations is now possible in most people with rheumatoid arthritis.

From a medical standpoint, when it comes to treating rheumatoid arthritis you could say that "the times, they are a-changin'." Doctors have a much better understanding of the whole disease process. This has led to the evolution of new treatment strategies with more effective medications. The goal? To quickly control inflammation, preserving the ability to move easily and reducing the joint damage once commonly seen in people with rheumatoid arthritis.

Many advances in the drug treatment of rheumatoid arthritis have been seen over the last 15 years, including introduction of new drugs, new ways of using old drugs and recognition that combinations of drugs may be more helpful than one drug at a time. These developments make the outlook for people with rheumatoid arthritis much better than at any time since the disease was first described. Although there have been no miracles, scientists and doctors have worked

steadily toward better understanding and better treatments with many important advances. In this chapter, we will review some of the principles of drug therapy for rheumatoid arthritis. In the chapter that follows, we will discuss the drugs themselves.

Acute vs. Chronic Disease

You may remember that in Chapter 1 we discussed some of the differences between acute and chronic diseases. These differences are most apparent when it comes to treatment strategies. With an *acute illness*, there is often a set protocol or treatment to be followed. For example, when a person has an acute infection, most of the decisions – including which drugs to take, when to take them and what other measures are necessary – are made by doctors, nurses and other health professionals. A laboratory test is used to identify an appropriate antibiotic. Even if the acute disease is severe and life-threatening, the outcome typically is known within a week or two.

Many acute diseases are self-limited, such as the common cold or a mild musculoskeletal sports injury. Drugs may cure these, hasten the recovery process or simply make a person feel better.

With a *chronic illness*, things are very different. Treatment cannot be regarded as a *cure*, but rather as a means to *control* symptoms and *prevent* damage. Although recommendations regarding which drugs to take and when to take them are made by doctors, nurses and other health professionals, the implementation of these decisions lies in the domain of the patient. The outcome may not be known for 10 to 20 years. A person with chronic disease has a great deal more control over his or her own management than a person with an acute illness. If you have rheumatoid arthritis, you become, in a sense, your own case manager.

One Drug vs. Many Drugs

Another concept to recognize is the distinction between diseases for which a single "best" drug can be identified and diseases in which there are many different "best" drugs. Again, many of our ideas about the treatment of diseases are derived from the treatment of an infectious disease. In an infectious disease, we sometimes forget that although a person may appear to be cured by taking an antibiotic, the target of the antibiotic is not the person, but rather a specific microorganism. In this setting, a drug that works in one person is likely to work equally well in other people with the same infection, taking into consideration that some people may have allergic reactions to certain drugs and may need an alternative treatment. It is usually possible to identify the best drug for a given infection.

In treating rheumatoid arthritis, people are complex and differ from one another in genetic makeup, levels of nutrition and many other factors that may affect the choice of drug. There is no single best drug for all people with rheumatoid arthritis, although there is evidence that certain drugs are better in more people than other drugs. Naming the best drug for all people with rheumatoid arthritis is a little like trying to name the best flavor of ice cream for all people. The best-selling flavor might be preferred by most people, but there will always be some people who like another flavor better.

The Traditional Approach to Medical Management

The medical approach to treating rheumatoid arthritis, as well as other chronic diseases, is based on a principle to "do no harm." That is, the treatment prescribed should not be worse than the disease itself. This remains a valid principle in any type of medical care – *as long as the judgment of what is harmful is based on a realistic assessment of how harmful the disease might be.*

In the traditional approach, sometimes called the pyramid approach, doctors were concerned that many of the drugs might be more harmful to people than the rheumatoid arthritis. Doctors started at the base of the pyramid with first-line drugs, such as nonsteroidal anti-inflammatory drugs (NSAIDs) or salicylates (such as aspirin), along with simple measures such as patient education and physical therapy. If these medicines did not control the disease, doc-

tors then moved up the pyramid to the more powerful disease-modifying and immunosuppressive drugs. Progressing up the pyramid could take quite a while, because the effectiveness of many of the drugs cannot be determined until after a considerable period of time – sometimes even several months.

The problem with applying this approach to rheumatoid arthritis was that, in the past, doctors did not have a complete understanding of the disease process or the amount of joint damage that could result in the first few years of this chronic condition. Research has shown that in the first two years of persistent arthritis, joint damage is likely to have already begun. Once these factors were understood, the strategy of treatment changed and doctors

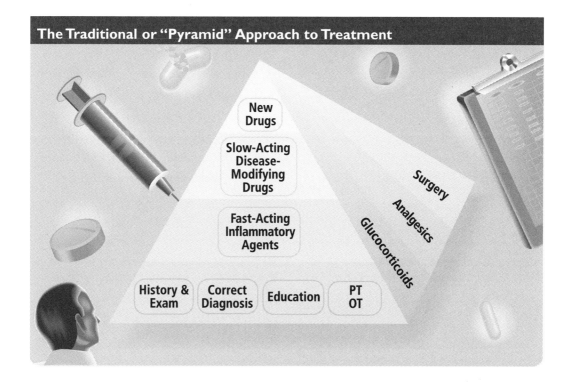

The Traditional or "Pyramid" Approach to Treatment

New Drugs

Slow-Acting Disease-Modifying Drugs

Surgery

Analgesics

Fast-Acting Inflammatory Agents

Glucocorticoids

History & Exam

Correct Diagnosis

Education

PT OT

began prescribing more powerful medicines earlier in the course of the disease.

Another problem with the traditional approach to treatment is that some of the older drugs, such as gold injections and penicillamine, have a much higher likelihood of side effects than newer drugs, such as methotrexate. The newer drugs have allowed more aggressive approaches to the management of rheumatoid arthritis.

The New Approach: A Preventive Strategy

At this time, doctors attempt to use powerful drugs early in the disease course in an effort to control inflammation and prevent damage to joints. This approach may be regarded as similar to early, aggressive treatment of high blood pressure to prevent long-term damage to the heart and blood vessels. There is no point in hiding the fact that rheumatoid arthritis can lead to severe long-term outcomes. By recognizing and even emphasizing the possible damage to the body that may result from a disease, doctors, other health professionals, patients, and their friends and families may be mobilized to act to prevent these consequences.

This approach to prevention has made a big difference in cardiovascular disease and is beginning to make a big difference in rheumatoid arthritis. Early inflammation, which is seen as joint swelling and tenderness, can be reversed and does not necessarily lead to damage if it is treated effectively.

Once there is damage, which is seen as physical joint malalignment and X-ray changes, it is probably not reversible. However, drug treatment can stop further damage.

Modern treatment of rheumatoid arthritis involves early use of powerful drugs. Combinations of these drugs are used by most specialists in rheumatology. In fact, most people must take at least two drugs to adequately control disease, and many people take three or four different drugs.

Is This New Approach Safe?

The traditional approach to treating rheumatoid arthritis was slow and often produced disappointing results. In addition, some of the drugs thought to be less harmful actually had fairly severe side effects. But what about these new strategies? Are they really more effective? And are they safe?

It's true that evidence is still incomplete on the effects of taking several drugs — especially the powerful, disease-modifying ones — in combination to treat rheumatoid arthritis. There is the possibility they could be more toxic than each drug taken alone. However, research studies indicate that combinations of drugs are no more likely to cause side effects than drugs taken individually. Aggressive therapy, including drug combinations, has the very real potential to minimize joint damage that previously occurred during the early years of disease in some people. And of course, as always, you must keep in mind that different people have different responses to these medications. Some individuals will do just fine with a conservative approach, but others will obviously need the more aggressive treatment strategies.

The issue is really not so much "Is my disease so bad that I need the aggressive treatment?" but rather, "Can I be better off in five years with aggressive treatment?" It is now known that the "side effects" of rheumatoid arthritis are considerably worse than the side effects of many of the drugs used to treat the disease.

What You Can Do

Learning about the drugs your doctor prescribes, how they work, the benefits and their potential side effects is the most important thing you can do. By alerting your doctor early to signs of a particular side effect, your medication can be reduced or changed as appropriate. Also, be sure to take your medication according to the doctor's instructions because this can help prevent, or minimize, side effects.

Rheumatoid arthritis takes a different course in each person. So your specific needs and reactions to the drugs may differ from those of others with the disease. It is *your* needs and reactions that your doctor will consider first when developing or changing your treatment program.

Personally Speaking Stories from real people with rheumatoid arthritis

"**E**very morning, it is a chore to grab my glasses. It hurts to walk across the ceramic tile in the bathroom. I drop things all morning while I'm getting ready.

"Although the pain is largely under control with drugs, it's the small things that never let me forget the disease. During high school and college, I was a celebrity, or at the very least, a conversation piece. Most kids that age don't know anyone with arthritis. It was harder once I entered the real world. The real world doesn't wait for a sore wrist or a limp. This was very hard for me to accept. I finally decided that the change had to be in me.

There Is No Time in My Life for Self-Pity
by Danielle Baker, Bedford, TX

"There is no time in my life for self-pity. I work 40-60 hours a week, have been married for four months, have a beautiful home and wonderful family and friends. I made up my mind to focus on these things, the parts of my life that are good. After all, I can walk, even run on occasion, although with a slight limp. I can still type and write, even with a deformed hand. I now make a point to park away from doors, and to attempt activities on my own before asking for help. There may be a day when I can't walk or write, but it is not today!"

Stopping Drug Treatment

If you feel much better after taking medications, you may be tempted to discontinue drug therapy because you feel so good. Stopping the therapy may be all right for a few weeks or even months. However, in most patients, a relapse is almost inevitable, usually within several weeks or months. In addition, getting the disease back under control will often be more difficult. It may be hard for you to continue to take drugs when there is no evidence of disease, but that generally seems to be the most desirable course. It is a little like the need for a person with diabetes to continue taking insulin to control blood sugar. The best strategy is to keep things as normal as possible to prevent damage, which includes giving treatment when there is no evidence of the condition.

"ASK THE DOCTOR" Worksheet

Complete This Part Before The Visit

1. What is the main reason I am going to the doctor?

   _____

   _____

2. Is there anything else that concerns me about my health or treatment (e.g., effect of rheumatoid arthritis on work, family or mood; problems following the recommended treatment plan)? _____Yes_____No

   _____

3. What do I want the doctor to do today?

   _____

   _____

4. The symptoms that bother me the most are ... (What? Where? When did they start? Do they change over time? How long do they last?). NOTE: bring copies of any completed self-monitoring forms/diaries.

   _____

   _____

5. What medications (prescriptions and over-the-counter) am I taking regularly? (List name(s) and dosage or take the bottles to your appointment.)

   _____

   _____

6. What are my goals for treatment (what I want or expect to get out of treatment)?

   _____

   _____

7. Prepare and prioritize a list of questions to give the doctor early in the visit.

   _____

   _____

   _____

8. Do I need Medicare, Medicaid or other insurance cards/forms today? _____Yes _____ No

   _____

"ASK THE DOCTOR" Worksheet

Questions to ask your doctor during the visit.

1. What is happening to me? How is my rheumatoid arthritis likely to affect me?

   _____

   _____

2. What are the results of my tests and what do they mean? May I have a copy of the results?

   _____

3. Why do I need the lab tests or X-rays that you are recommending today?

   _____

4. Are there any risks from these tests?

   _____

5. When should I call for the results?

   _____

6. What should I do at home (diet, activity, treatment options, special instructions, medications, precautions, etc.)?

   _____

   _____

   a. What are the benefits, costs and drawbacks (or risks) for each option for treatment?

   _____

   b. How and how often do I do the treatment? _____

   c. How long should I give it a try? _____

   _____

7. When should I call if my condition doesn't get better and the treatment does not seem to be working? What additional symptoms would warrant my calling before my next scheduled visit?

   _____

   _____

8. When should I return for another visit?

   _____

"ASK THE DOCTOR" Worksheet

Medication questions:

1. What is the name of the drug?_____

2. What are the purpose and benefits of this drug?

   _____

3. How quickly does it work? How long should I take this drug?

   _____

4. What are the possible side effects or drawbacks to the drug?

   _____

   a. When should I contact you about side effects?

   _____

   b. What can I do to prevent or deal with the side effects or drawbacks?

   _____

5. Is it all right to take the drug with other drugs (such as cold, sinus, allergy, pain medicines)
   I am taking? _____Yes _____No
   If not, what drugs should I avoid? _____

   _____

6. When is the best time to take the drug? Before, with or after meals? _____

7. What should I do if I forget to take my medicine?

   _____

8. Are there any changes I should make in my diet? _____Yes _____No
   If so, what?_____

   a. Can I drink alcohol while taking this drug? _____Yes _____No

   b. Are there any other restrictions? _____Yes _____No
   If so, what?_____

9. Should I avoid driving or any other activity while taking this drug? _____Yes _____No

10. Is a generic drug available? If so, is the generic form as effective? _____Yes _____No

Chapter 11

Aggressive Therapy:

Medications and Treatments for Rheumatoid Arthritis

Living well with rheumatoid arthritis involves a great deal of self-management activities including diet, exercise and dealing positively with stress. But the most important component of treatment of rheumatoid arthritis is medication, and a number of new, effective drugs have emerged in recent years. In this chapter we will review the specific types of drugs that are used for rheumatoid arthritis. First, we'll define the different categories of drugs in brief.

NONSTEROIDAL ANTI-INFLAMMATORY DRUGS (NSAIDs)

Nonsteroidal anti-inflammatory drugs or NSAIDs are drugs similar to aspirin that can reduce inflammation. In reducing inflammation, these drugs also relieve pain. There are three generations of these drugs. The first is aspirin, which, in its non-coated form, is often irritating to the stomach. The second generation is other forms of aspirin (such as enteric-coated and zero-order release aspirin) and drugs such as ibuprofen (*Motrin, Advil*), naproxen (*Naprosyn, Aleve*), indomethacin (*Indocin*) and others. These are often as effective as aspirin, but with less irritation of the stomach. Most recently, a third generation of NSAIDs known as COX-2 inhibitors, including celecoxib (*Celebrex*) and rofecoxib (*Vioxx*), has been developed. These drugs have even greater safety from gastrointestinal events and are discussed more extensively later in this chapter.

ANALGESIC DRUGS

Analgesic drugs are those designed specifically to relieve pain without necessarily having an effect on inflammation. The prototype drug in this class is acetaminophen (*Tylenol*), which may be combined with other pain-relieving drugs such as codeine. Another widely used analgesic drug is propoxyphene (*Darvon*). In addition, there are stronger narcotic analgesic drugs such as meperidine (*Demerol*), morphine, and compounds such as *Percocet, Percodan, Vicodin* and others.

GLUCOCORTICOIDS OR PREDNISONE

Glucocorticoids are naturally occurring compounds required by the body for carrying out normal life processes. When cortisone was first given to people with rheumatoid arthritis in 1948, it was thought to be a miracle drug and perhaps even the cure for the disease. Unfortunately, cortisone or prednisone – the most commonly used chemical form of cortisone – caused many serious side effects that often became worse than the disease itself. From the 1950s through the 1980s, doctors recommended that cortisone or prednisone not be used at all in rheumatoid arthritis, except for treating the most severe complications. However, over the last 15 years it has been recognized that low doses of cortisone, such as 5 mg of prednisone or less, can be taken reasonably safely over long periods to prevent joint damage without introducing major side effects.

METHOTREXATE

The most important disease-modifying antirheumatic drug, or DMARD, introduced for the care of rheumatoid arthritis over the last 20 years has been methotrexate (*Rheumatrex)*. Disease-modifying antirheumatic drugs appear to have the capacity to slow joint destruction in rheumatoid arthritis over time. Methotrexate is presently taken by more than one half of people with rheumatoid arthritis treated in the United States at this time.

OTHER DMARDS

Disease-modifying antirheumatic drugs are used in addition to nonsteroidal anti-inflammatory drugs and prednisone. The most important DMARD is methotrexate, as noted previously. The classic DMARD is injectable gold, which is still quite effective in some people. Other DMARDs include penicillamine (*Depen*), azathioprine (*Imuran*) and chloroquine. Over the last 20 years, hydroxychloroquine (*Plaquenil*), sulfasalazine (*Azulfidine*), and oral gold (*Ridaura*) have been introduced. Another drug currently used to treat rheumatoid arthritis, although not technically a DMARD, is minocycline (*Minocin*).

IMMUNOMODULATING DRUGS AND APPROACHES

In the 1990s, at least five drugs and devices that directly modify the immune system have been introduced, including cyclosporine (*Neoral*), leflunomide (*Arava*), etanercept (*Enbrel*), the *Prosorba* column and infliximab (*Remicade*). Cyclosporine and leflunomide are chemical compounds that modify immune function and are often very effective in controlling rheumatoid arthritis symptoms. Etanercept and infliximab are the first of a class of drugs that specifically inhibit chemicals that are involved in the inflammatory response. The *Prosorba* column removes certain antibodies associated with rheumatoid arthritis through a chemical and mechanical filtering process.

Nonsteroidal Anti-Inflammatory Drugs (NSAIDs)

Nonsteroidal anti-inflammatory drugs (NSAIDs) are a family of drugs that reduce (and sometimes even eliminate) inflammation, and thereby lessen pain in people with rheumatoid arthritis. Joint inflammation results from the production of certain chemicals called *cytokines*, which, in turn, stimulate a subgroup of chemicals called prostaglandins. A primary action of NSAIDs is to inhibit production of prostaglandins, which reduces the inflammation and pain associated with rheumatoid arthritis.

As we discussed in Chapter 2, the inflammatory response normally serves to protect the body from invasion by an infection or bacterium, and to help heal wounds such as a cut or fracture. When the inflammatory process has accomplished its mission, the production of its chemicals is "turned off" through complex control mechanisms.

When regulated properly, prostaglandins and cytokines are not in the body to be harmful, but to protect us. However, the signals to turn off the process are not controlled properly in people with rheumatoid arthritis. Prostaglandins and cytokines are produced when they shouldn't be, leading to inflammation, pain and long-term damage.

In addition to their role in the normal inflammatory response, prostaglandins are also normally found in certain tissues and organs to perform necessary functions. For example, prostaglandins help protect the lining of the stomach from acid, which can eat away at the stomach and cause bleeding or a hole in the stomach called an ulcer. Because NSAIDs reduce the production of prostaglandins, they may cause stomach irritation and undesirable gastrointestinal side effects. Prostaglandins also aid in removal of fluid from the kidneys, maintain a balance of competing chemicals in the brain, and promote normal blood clotting in platelets. That is why NSAIDs may cause problems with kidney function, such as fluid retention, or with the central nervous system function, such as headaches and feeling "spacey." NSAIDs may also interfere with normal blood clotting, which is the reason surgeons ask patients to stop taking NSAIDs for a week or two prior to surgery. Fortunately, some of the newer NSAIDs are associated with fewer of these types of problems, as will be discussed below.

ASPIRIN: THE CLASSIC NSAID

Aspirin has been used as a medicine since ancient times. Long ago, people realized that eating the bark of the willow tree, or drinking a tea brewed from the bark, could be helpful for some illnesses. In the late 19th century, the active chemical in willow bark (called *salicylate*) was synthesized as a pill.

Aspirin remains a very effective drug for relief of inflammation and pain. However, plain aspirin is too irritating to the stomach for long-term use in the high quantities needed for treating rheumatoid arthritis.

Other forms of aspirin including *Ascriptin* (aspirin mixed with *Maalox*), enteric-coated aspirin (*Ecotrin*) and zero-order release aspirin (*ZORprin*) have been created that lead to much lower levels of stomach irritation. Even when aspirin is not absorbed in the stomach (for instance, when it is given as a suppository through the rectum or as a zero-order release aspirin absorbed in the small intestine), some stomach irritation occurs, indicating that general systemic effects of aspirin lead to stomach irritation.

Research studies show that the newer, less irritating forms of aspirin are favored by more people with rheumatoid arthritis than any of the other NSAIDs available before 1990. There is still a place for aspirin and its analogs in the treatment of certain people with rheumatoid arthritis.

OTHER TRADITIONAL NSAIDS

Beginning in the 1970s, a number of other NSAIDs were developed by the pharmaceutical industry. Indomethacin (*Indocin*) and ibuprofen (*Motrin, Advil, Nuprin*) were among the first non-aspirin forms developed. These anti-inflammatory drugs did not have the same chemical composition as aspirin, and many people found them easier to take. These NSAIDs carried with them the same potential side effects as aspirin – irritation of the stomach, interference with removal of fluid by the kidneys, imbalance in the central nervous system and reduced blood clotting – although at lower levels.

Indomethacin is usually not very helpful to most people with rheumatoid arthritis, although a few people experience great benefit. Indomethacin may cause unacceptable headaches and "spacey" feelings in more people than any other NSAID. Nonetheless, every person is different – one of the recurring themes of this book – so if only two percent of people with rheumatoid arthritis benefit substantially from indomethacin use, that drug is well worth trying for those few people.

Ibuprofen was the first major alternative to aspirin. Many people who take ibuprofen experience as much pain relief as with aspirin, but have less gastrointestinal discomfort. In addition, there is a lower risk of severe gastrointestinal irritation and events than with aspirin. Ibuprofen is the most widely-used NSAID, particularly since 1992 when it became available over the counter as *Advil, Nuprin, Motrin* or *Mediprin*. The nonprescription 200-mg dose is often not sufficient for people with rheumatoid arthritis, although it may be quite effective for a relatively minor trauma such as a strained muscle. People with rheumatoid arthritis often need 400, 600 or even 800 mg of ibuprofen several times a day to gain effective pain relief.

One drawback to the use of ibuprofen, aspirin and other traditional NSAIDs is that they must be taken at least three or four times per day to give people the best benefit, because their effects only last for a few hours. This problem led scientists to develop longer-acting NSAIDs, which only need to be taken twice or even once per day. Some of the more widely used long-acting NSAIDs include naproxen (*Naprosyn*), which is available in doses of 250, 375 and 500 mg, and also is available without a prescription as *Aleve* in a dose of 220 mg. Other twice-a-day compounds include nabumetone (*Relafen*), ketoprofen (*Orudis, Oruvail*) and diclofenac sodium (*Voltaren*). Indomethacin also comes in a slow-release form for twice-daily usage (*Indocin SR*). Some of the once-a-day NSAIDs include piroxicam (*Feldene*) and oxaprozin (*Daypro*). Although these newer NSAIDs are taken less frequently, they still have the same potential

gastrointestinal side effects of NSAIDs. Details concerning these drugs are found in the table at the end of this chapter, which reviews many of the drugs currently used to treat rheumatoid arthritis.

THE GASTROINTESTINAL DILEMMA

The problem of gastrointestinal irritation was recognized in the 1980s as a major problem in the use of NSAIDs in all forms of arthritis. Several types of research studies indicated that every year about one of every 50 to 100 people who took an NSAID regularly would experience a major gastrointestinal event, such as bleeding ulcer or perforation, leading to hospitalization. One in 50

Personally Speaking — Stories from real people with rheumatoid arthritis

"There was a smile on my face today as I woke up. I stretched and greeted my day. My mind rehearsed all the things I was going to get done. Wow, was I excited!

"I commanded my body to get up onto my feet, but not without my two best friends by my side: Can and Will, my crutches. My eyes start to flood with tears at the realization that no miracle has happened overnight.

Can and Will: My Two Best Friends
by Angelica Molloy, Salt Lake City, UT

"The excruciating pain that hits as I maneuver each foot slowly subsides to a tolerable degree. Now, I look forward to my warm shower. Allowing the gentle flow of the water to comfort my aching body, I wish I could scrub myself to a newborn clean.

"My next adventure is dressing. That means pulling, tugging, bending and buttoning. Breakfast means walking, reaching, opening and cooking. I haven't done much, but already, I'm exhausted.

"So how do I make it through the day and cope with these seemingly small frustrations that can leave me crying? I make it to my typewriter. There, I unload my feelings into my journal, or into poetry."

to 100 people may not sound like a lot of people, but if millions of people take these drugs, then thousands of people could expect to have serious side effects from the use of NSAIDs.

One important matter concerning NSAID-related gastrointestinal side effects is that a person might experience an acute problem such as internal bleeding, a hole or perforation, or an obstruction in the stomach without any warning signs or symptoms such as pain, nausea or heartburn. By contrast, other people may have many symptoms and never experience a serious gastrointestinal event. Although patients and doctors respond primarily to symptoms – that is, reports of heartburn or stomach pain – the major reason to be concerned about the gastrointestinal tract may not be pain, but risk of a serious event. This risk increases substantially in people over age 75, those with a previous history of gastrointestinal events and those with more active, severe joint disease.

The risk of serious gastrointestinal events prevents many people from taking the traditional NSAIDs. With earlier use of disease-modifying antirheumatic drugs (DMARDs), as we discussed in Chapter 10, NSAIDs are no longer regarded as the mainstay of the treatment of rheumatoid arthritis. Nonetheless, more than 60 percent of patients continue to take these drugs, more for their ability to relieve pain than for their anti-inflammatory activity. In addition, NSAIDs are widely used for treating other

rheumatic conditions including osteoarthritis and bursitis, among others. Because of their continued usefulness, here are four strategies for reducing the gastrointestinal side effects of NSAIDs by using other drugs to protect the stomach.

• **Antacid drugs.** The first strategy involves the addition of drugs that might protect the lining of the stomach. One of the early attempts was a combination of aspirin and *Maalox* (*Ascriptin*), which many people found to cause less gastrointestinal irritation than plain aspirin. There was still a substantial rate of gastrointestinal ulcers and irritation, however, apparently due to the fact that aspirin could still be irritating to the stomach. This strategy helped alleviate some symptoms, but it did not necessarily reduce the risk of serious events.

• **H2 blockers.** During the 1970s, a new class of compounds was developed called H2 blockers. These agents included cimetidine (*Tagamet*), famotidine (*Pepcid*), ranitidine (*Zantac*) and nizatidine (*Axid*). H2 blockers act by blocking receptors in the stomach that lead to the production of acid. The net result is less acid production. There is some reduction of the gastrointestinal irritation associated with NSAIDs with these drugs, but the protection provided by H2 blockers is far from complete.

• **Prostaglandin combinations.** Researchers have developed a pill that contains a synthetic prostaglandin called misoprostol (*Cytotec*). When taken with an NSAID, it helps to protect the stomach locally from irritation. Recently, a drug that contains diclofenac sodium (*Voltaren*) coated with misoprostol has been developed (*Arthrotec*). *Arthrotec* can be taken twice per day, and many people have found this to be a very effective drug.

• **Proton pump inhibitors.** More recently, a class of gastrointestinal compounds known as *proton pump inhibitors* has become available that often provides even more effective relief than H2 blockers. Examples include omeprazole (*Prilosec*) and lansoprazole (*Prevacid*). Studies have documented that proton pump inhibitors can protect the stomach against the gastrointestinal side effects associated with NSAIDs because they block the secretion of acid into the stomach more effectively than H2 blockers.

COX-2 INHIBITORS

During the 1990s, it was discovered that two types of enzymes called cyclooxygenase enzymes, or COX enzymes, lead to the synthesis of prostaglandins. Cyclooxygenase-1 (COX-1) is associated with many of the "healthy" functions of prostaglandins, such as protecting the lining of the stomach, helping to remove fluids, maintaining balance in the central nervous system and promoting blood clotting. Cyclooxygenase-2 (COX-2) is associated with some other functions of prostaglandins, including the inflammatory response. In theory, a drug that inhibits COX-2 but not COX-1 would be able to inhibit the inflammatory response that occurs in rheumatoid arthritis without

having the undesirable effects of some of the traditional NSAIDs, particularly the possibility of irritating the stomach and causing gastrointestinal events such as bleeding and perforation of the stomach.

Two selective COX-2 inhibitors are currently available on the market. They are known as celecoxib (*Celebrex*) and rofecoxib (*Vioxx*).

DO NSAIDS HAVE A ROLE IN THE FUTURE?

The role of NSAIDs in rheumatoid arthritis is being reassessed. Previously it was suggested that NSAIDs should be used in all patients as the first line of therapy. However, with the availability of powerful, new disease-modifying antirheumatic drugs (DMARDs), NSAIDs may not be needed in some people.

Many doctors are now using NSAIDs primarily for their analgesic (pain-relieving) properties. These drugs are able to relieve pain over and above their capacity to relieve inflammation. Very few people with rheumatoid arthritis are treated with NSAIDs alone now, because of evidence that NSAIDs alone are not sufficient to block the progression of joint destruction and functional disability. Instead, they may be used in combination with DMARDs to achieve the best possible control of pain and inflammation.

Analgesic Drugs

Analgesic drugs relieve pain without necessarily having any effect on inflammation.

Their effectiveness stems from the fact that they act on the brain or the central nervous system, which is where pain is perceived. As discussed in Chapter 2, it is generally better for pain to be relieved by controlling inflammation through the use of anti-inflammatory drugs. However, in certain patients at certain times – and in people who have painful joints as a result of joint damage, but no longer have active inflammation – it is often helpful to use drugs specifically to relieve pain. Furthermore, people may need pain relief for a specific event such as extraction of a tooth or menstrual pain over and above their usual arthritis medications.

PAIN: IT'S ALL IN YOUR HEAD

Sometimes people confronted with severe pain may ask, "Is all of this pain in my head?" Well, the correct answer is that all pain *is* experienced in the head, although it may reflect problems in an arm or leg. For example, if you have a fractured leg that needs to be manipulated, you are given anesthesia and put to sleep, at which point there is no more pain. This is an important principle, because it reminds us that the perception of pain can be greater or lesser depending, in part, on how it is interpreted in the brain.

Sometimes pain cannot be explained by inflammation or structural changes. This common form of musculoskeletal pain is experienced by people who have fibromyalgia. People with rheumatoid arthritis may also have fibromyalgia, as discussed in Chapter 5, and may require additional therapy.

ACETAMINOPHEN (*TYLENOL*)

The most widely-used analgesic drug in the United States is acetaminophen, which is also known as paracetamol (*Panadol)* in Europe. It is available over-the-counter in doses of 325 mg or 500 mg.

Acetaminophen is often thought of as a substitute for NSAIDs. It may be a good substitute for some people when it comes to reducing fever or relieving pain, but acetaminophen is not a good substitute with respect to the reduction of inflammation, one of the primary actions of aspirin. There is a slight reduction of inflammation associated with the use of acetaminophen, but it is very minimal compared with aspirin. So although you can substitute acetaminophen for aspirin when you have a headache or a toothache, you cannot substitute acetaminophen for aspirin for the inflammation in rheumatoid arthritis. At the least, it will not have the same potential value as an anti-inflammatory drug.

Acetaminophen is now recommended as the first drug to be used for the pain of osteoarthritis, which in effect is what a person with rheumatoid arthritis who has damaged joints may be experiencing. Acetaminophen may be helpful when pain is not the result of inflammation in a person who might have damage to joints from long-standing rheumatoid arthritis.

Acetaminophen is often combined with a narcotic. Most frequently it is mixed with codeine as *Tylenol* #1, 2, 3 or 4, containing 15, 30, 45 and 60 mg of codeine, respectively. This combination is used by doctors for conditions that may cause pain beyond that of the rheumatoid arthritis or to "tide over" somebody during a flare of disease activity. Acetaminophen as a single drug or as a compound is usually *not* an effective long-term drug to be used for treating rheumatoid arthritis.

NARCOTIC DRUGS

A number of narcotic drugs are used as pain relievers. In general, these drugs relieve pain more effectively than anti-inflammatory drugs or non-narcotic analgesic drugs. They include codeine, meperidine (*Demerol*), propoxyphene (*Darvon*), morphine, oxycodone, hydrocodone (*Vicodin*) and tramadol (*Ultram*). These drugs are often used in combination with acetaminophen and other drugs.

A general rule of thumb in treating rheumatoid arthritis or other rheumatic diseases has been to avoid the use of narcotic drugs under any conditions. Although it is true that one should think twice about the use of narcotic drugs, this position has been slowly modified just as the position about prednisone and other drugs has been modified. It is now believed that many people may benefit from the judicious use of narcotic drugs. Although there is a certain danger of addiction to narcotic drugs, studies have shown that people who experience severe pain are unlikely to become addicted – in contrast to people who have no pain and take narcotic drugs for other types of effects on the brain.

Different doctors have very different views of the use of narcotic drugs. In general, research studies show that doctors tend to underestimate pain experienced by their patients, leading to "undermedication" by the doctor and frustration of the patient. The use of questionnaires with pain scores has been very helpful in documenting the severity of pain from a patient's perspective, and many doctors use these measures in routine care to judge the need for additional pain relief.

A number of narcotic compounds are available to treat pain. We emphasize that these are not intended for long-term use, but for occasional use in flares or other events that might occur, most likely from a fracture or other severe acute event. These drugs include *Percodan*, *Percocet* and *Lortab*. Some narcotic compounds can be given in the form of a patch worn on the skin, such as the *Duragesic* patch. This form of the drug may be helpful in certain situations, such as when a person experiences a compression fracture of the spine, which can be acutely painful but that heals over time without long-term consequences.

One simple analgesic drug that has been used extensively is propoxyphene (*Darvon*). This drug's effectiveness in relieving pain has been shown to be comparable to acetaminophen in the population. As with all drugs, however, some people find propoxyphene more effective than acetaminophen, just as other people may find acetaminophen more effective than propoxyphene.

Glucocorticoids (Cortisone, Prednisone)

Probably no drugs used in the treatment of rheumatoid arthritis, or even in clinical medicine in general, evoke more controversy than glucocorticoids. These are a group of hormones that are produced naturally by the *adrenal gland*, an internal organ situated above the kidney. In the body, glucocorticoids help support the circulatory system and regulate body functions. All of us make about 25 mg to 35 mg of cortisol (our naturally occurring glucocorticoid) each day to support vital body functions. All humans need a certain level of glucocorticoids to sustain life itself.

An important drug in the treatment of rheumatoid arthritis is prednisone, a synthetically produced version of cortisone. Synthetically produced cortisone is roughly similar to cortisol in its activity as a glucocorticoid. On the other hand, prednisone is about five times more powerful than cortisone – which means that 25–35 mg of cortisone are roughly equivalent to 5–7 mg of prednisone. Prednisone also comes in an injectable form called *Depo-Medrol* and *Solu-Medrol*. The most powerful glucocorticoid is dexamethasone, which is about 10 times more powerful than cortisone, so that 25 mg of cortisone is equivalent to 2.5 mg of dexamethasone.

A number of serious side effects may occur when people take high doses of glucocorticoids over long periods. These include weight gain, "moon face" appearance, increased susceptibility to infection, diabetes, high blood pressure, cataracts, avascular necrosis of the hip and other bones, and osteoporosis (thinning of bones). There is also a naturally occurring human condition called Cushing's syndrome or hyperadrenocorticism, in which too much cortisol is made due to a dysregulation in the adrenal gland or due to a hormone-producing tumor. People with this condition may develop the same serious symptoms as people who take high doses of glucocorticoids over long periods.

HIGH-DOSE VS. LOW-DOSE GLUCOCORTICOIDS

One of the functions of glucocorticoids is to shut down the inflammatory response after it is no longer needed to protect the body from infections or other events that may "jump start" the immune system (see Chapter 2).

Glucocorticoids such as cortisone or prednisone may be prescribed to treat a variety of inflammatory conditions ranging from an acute insect bite or poison ivy to serious rheumatic diseases like rheumatoid arthritis or systemic lupus. For certain conditions, such as an attack of asthma, high doses such as 20–60 mg of prednisone are given, often in a "*dose-pack*." In this form, the amount of glucocorticoid is tapered down over the course of a week to treat subacute inflammatory conditions. Of course, people generally recover from these conditions, but the glucocorticoids may hasten the recovery, make recovery more likely, or even save the person's life. Regardless, the action of the glucocorticoids is needed over only a few days.

When high-dose glucocorticoids are used in a chronic condition such as rheumatoid arthritis, the situation becomes more complex. One reason is that the inflammation stimulus continues rather than disappears. If the glucocorticoid dose is tapered rapidly, as in a dose-pack, symptoms tend to return when the dose reaches a low level or the drug is discontinued. There may even be a strong "rebound" effect in which symptoms actually increase. Occasionally, some physicians use high doses of pills or an injection of glucocorticoids that are then rapidly tapered to normal levels to control acute flares. But over long periods, an effort is made to maintain dosage at less than 5 mg of prednisone per day.

Most people with rheumatoid arthritis appear to respond to low doses of glucocorticoids (such as 5 mg or less of prednisone) similar to those made naturally in the adrenal gland. The side effects of long-term, low-dose glucocorticoid use are much less serious than those seen with high doses. Side effects may still be seen – thinning of the skin, easy bruising and poorer wound healing, for example – but most of the major consequences, such as diabetes, hypertension and weight gain, are only slightly or no more common than in the general population of people with chronic diseases.

Many rheumatoid arthritis specialists suggest that the capacity of low-dose glucocorti-coids to help people function from day to day, relieve pain and slow long-term joint damage makes their use worthwhile.

HISTORY OF USE OF GLUCOCORTICOIDS IN RHEUMATOID ARTHRITIS

Cortisone was first produced in the laboratory in 1948. It was immediately apparent that cortisone could lead to major benefit in people with rheumatoid arthritis and other inflammatory conditions. The effects of cortisone appeared almost as a "miracle" in the improvement seen overnight in many people. Magazine articles in the popular press at the time described the dramatic effects of cortisone, and many believed there was finally a cure for rheumatoid arthritis.

This period of great hope lasted only a few years. By the early 1950s, it was recognized that high doses of glucocorticoids over periods longer than a few weeks or months were associated with severe side effects. The consequences often appeared to be as bad as, or even worse than, the disease itself. The medical community concluded that it would be undesirable to use *any* glucocorticoids to treat rheumatoid arthritis. From the 1960s to the 1980s, medical texts recommended that these drugs be used only as a last resort if a person could not function at all or developed a severe consequence, such as vasculitis.

The medical community redefined its attitude on glucocorticoids in the 1980s, when it was recognized that low doses of these drugs could be used over long periods with fewer side effects than those seen with high doses. The idea was not to use high-dose glucocorticoids at all, but to prescribe them in low doses over long, even indefinite, periods. It was found that people could safely take prednisone in doses of 3 to 7.5 mg per day or less, which would yield most of the benefits of high doses with very few of the side effects. In 1992, it was found that 75 percent of people with rheumatoid arthritis under the care of rheumatologists in the United States were taking glucocorticoids, mostly over long periods and in low doses.

Of course, everyone is different. A few people experience psychological distress when they take *any* dose of glucocorticoids beyond what is naturally made in the body. These people can't take prednisone at all. However, benefits can be seen in doses as low as 1 mg per day.

DISCONTINUING GLUCOCORTICOIDS – SOME PRECAUTIONS

Long-term use of glucocorticoids in rheumatoid arthritis signals the body's adrenal glands to stop manufacturing cortisol. In such a case, were the person to experience an unusual stress, such as an accident or surgery, his or her body couldn't produce the boost of glucocorticoids needed. It would be necessary to give extra amounts of the drug. Likewise, a person who has taken high doses for more than a few weeks cannot abruptly stop taking them. A person may experience confusion and even collapse from not hav-

ing enough glucocorticoids if they are stopped suddenly. So you must taper the dose gradually while the adrenal glands, which make glucocorticoids in the body, build their capacity to produce normal amounts of cortisol. This process generally takes about a month or two.

GLUCOCORTICOIDS BY INJECTION

In addition to different types of glucocorticoid pills, these drugs may be given by injection in several ways. Four techniques are discussed briefly here.

• **A simple intramuscular injection.** An *intramuscular injection*, or a simple injection in a muscle, of a glucocorticoid may be given to quiet a generalized flare of rheumatoid arthritis. Two compounds often used for these injections are triamcinolone (*Kenalog*) and methylprednisolone (*Depo-Medrol*). Some people may be treated with intramuscular injections every two months rather than taking oral glucocorticoids. This type of injection often results in substantial benefit, which usually lasts from one to eight weeks. Any doctor or trained nurse can give an intramuscular injection.

• **Injection into a joint.** If a single joint is swollen out of proportion to other joints, it may be beneficial for a doctor to inject that joint directly with glucocorticoid, usually after removing as much fluid as possible (a process called *aspiration*). Joints commonly injected include the knees, ankles, shoulders, elbows, wrists and knuckles. This type of injection may be very effective to quiet inflammation in a specific joint. The injection delivers a much higher concentration of glucocorticoid directly into the joint, and does not expose you to the potential side effects of generalized glucocorticoids. Administration of an injection into a joint requires special training or experience.

- **Injection of glucocorticoids in soft tissues.** Glucocorticoid injections may be helpful for conditions such as tendinitis or bursitis (see Chapter 5) in which the site of inflammation involves the soft tissue near a joint, rather than the joint directly. For example, the drugs may be injected in the tissue around the wrist in people who have carpal tunnel syndrome, a condition in which there may be numbness and tingling in the fingers. A local glucocorticoid injection may also be given at the base of a finger to relieve a "trigger finger," in which a finger does not open up normally, but suddenly with a trigger action. Glucocorticoids may also be injected into tender points in people who have fibromyalgia along with rheumatoid arthritis (see Chapter 5).
- **Intravenous injection.** Intravenous glucocorticoid injections, sometimes in very high doses, are known as "pulses" (or "pulse therapy"). These pulses may be given in doses up to 1,000 mg, sometimes on three consecutive days. This treatment is effective but results are temporary, and many doctors think that low-dose, long-term glucocorticoids are just as helpful to people with rheumatoid arthritis. Since the introduction of many other effective treatments, the use of glucocorticoid pulses has declined considerably. However, this treatment may still be effective in certain situations.

GLUCOCORTICOIDS AS THE ONLY DRUG TREATMENT

Glucocorticoids may leave someone feeling so well that it may seem that there is no need for further medication. However, it is unusual that these drugs can be effective as the *only* treatment for most people with rheumatoid arthritis. In general, an additional drug, usually a disease-modifying antirheumatic drug (DMARD) – such as methotrexate, sulfasalazine, hydroxychloroquine or others – is needed.

WHAT SHOULD YOU WORRY ABOUT WHEN TAKING PREDNISONE?

The side effects listed for prednisone mostly are associated with high doses of this drug, and include higher likelihood of a "moon face," weight gain, hypertension, diabetes, osteoporosis and related fractures, and susceptibility to infections. Although these are not unusual in people who have taken *high* doses of glucocorticoids, they are quite unusual in most people who have taken *low* doses of prednisone, even over long periods. Many people have taken low-dose prednisone for more than 10 years and have normal bone densities. We must also remember that there is an increased likelihood of infection and osteoporosis associated with rheumatoid arthritis itself, which may be attributed to the glucocorticoid treatment but may be simply a manifestation of the disease.

Methotrexate

Methotrexate was first used in the 1940s to treat various forms of cancer, including leukemia and breast cancer. It was one of the first successful chemotherapy drugs. The main action of methotrexate in cancer is to kill cells that grow and divide without normal control mechanisms.

Rheumatoid arthritis is not a cancer, but there are cells in the joint that are not regulated normally. Therefore, the idea of killing abnormally dividing cells makes sense. There is a major difference in the strategy of killing cells in cancer compared to killing cells in arthritis, however. If 99 percent of the cancerous cells are killed, the 1 percent that survive usually will continue to divide and cause disease to return to its previous level. By contrast, in people with rheumatoid arthritis, if 80 percent of abnormal cells are killed, the patient usually becomes quite well, which is why much lower amounts of methotrexate are needed to treat rheumatoid arthritis – often less than one tenth as much as is used to treat cancer.

Although the original reason for using methotrexate to treat rheumatoid arthritis involved killing abnormal cells, it now seems likely that methotrexate works in rheumatoid arthritis primarily because of its activity against inflammation.

HIGH-DOSE AND LOW-DOSE METHOTREXATE

A simple example can help illustrate the difference between a small dose and a large dose of methotrexate: It's like the difference between a glass compared to a bottle of red wine. All bottles of wine have a warning that drinking the contents may be harmful to health, despite extensive evidence that one or two glasses a day are associated with living longer. However, one or two *bottles* a day of red wine is not associated with living longer, and in fact will probably shorten your life. Similarly, small doses of methotrexate may be quite safe and very beneficial, in contrast to large doses that are appropriate only for certain situations in people with cancer. (Similar considerations apply to prednisone, mentioned earlier in this chapter.)

High doses of methotrexate are associated with many severe side effects (including hair loss, mouth sores, decreased liver function and changes in blood counts) that can be dangerous and could leave a person more vulnerable to infection. By contrast, low doses cause changes in blood counts and liver function very infrequently, although some hair loss is not uncommon. Overall, low-dose methotrexate appears to be less likely to cause side effects than most drugs used in the treatment of rheumatoid arthritis, including many non-steroidal anti-inflammatory drugs.

ARE YOU A CANDIDATE FOR METHOTREXATE?

When methotrexate was first used in rheumatoid arthritis, it was reserved for people who had the most severe problems with long-standing disease. There was a great concern among doctors that the types of side effects we have discussed would not justify its use in people who had relatively mild disease. As might be expected, many of the people who were first treated with methotrexate had already experienced considerable joint damage. As we have discussed, medications may reduce or even eliminate inflammation entirely, but they cannot restore a joint to a normal state after it has been damaged over the years. Although there was substantial improvement in the people who had methotrexate treatment, most of them still experienced problems in functional disability and pain.

As long-term, widespread experience with methotrexate has been gained over the past 10 to 15 years, we now recognize that low-dose methotrexate has been the drug treatment most likely to control inflammation and prevent damage to joints. Some of the newer drugs, such as leflunomide (*Arava*), etanercept (*Enbrel*) and infliximab (*Remicade*) may be as effective as methotrexate, perhaps even more effective, in some people with rheumatoid arthritis.

As with all drugs, some people cannot take methotrexate. Nonetheless, with evidence of few side effects, which are manageable, methotrexate increasingly is used for *most* people with rheumatoid arthritis. Many doctors believe all people who have rheumatoid arthritis should take some dose of methotrexate if they can tolerate it. The most feared consequences of methotrexate – liver damage and impaired production of blood cells – are quite unusual when it is used in low doses.

WHEN SHOULD YOU BEGIN METHOTREXATE?

Here again, recommendations are changing. Traditionally, methotrexate was saved for later in the disease course. Now, with a goal of preventing damage, the drug is used early to treat inflammation as aggressively as possible. Of course, certain people may be candidates for other treatments, particularly as new, better and possibly safer drugs become available.

WHEN SHOULD METHOTREXATE BE DISCONTINUED?

Although all people prefer to discontinue drug treatment if possible, considerable evidence suggests that people who have responded to methotrexate and continue to tolerate it well should continue to take some dose on an indefinite basis. One hesitates to use the terms "forever" or "for life," because there is always a possibility that new and better treatments will be developed, or that the arthritis may remit. Medical research may some day find a drug that people need to take for only a few weeks or months rather than indefinitely. Until such treatments become available, however, the long-term use of methotrexate is one of the best ways for most people to control the inflammation of rheumatoid arthritis and prevent joint damage over many years.

WHEN SHOULD OTHER DRUGS BE ADDED?

Another matter that is changing rapidly involves the use of disease-modifying agents in combination to treat rheumatoid arthritis. It used to be that if you took a DMARD such as gold injections or penicillamine that seemed to work for a while and then seemed to stop working later, the doctor would discontinue that drug and begin another DMARD. Part of the reasoning was a concern that severe side effects were more likely if two powerful drugs were used together. But methotrexate has far fewer side effects than most of the other drugs used to treat rheumatoid arthritis. Therefore, it is now the practice among many doctors to add a second DMARD if methotrexate does not control swelling and pain entirely. "Combination therapy" with methotrexate and drugs such as hydroxychloroquine (*Plaquenil*), sulfasalazine (*Azulfidine*), etanercept (*Enbrel*), leflunomide (*Arava*) and infliximab (*Remicade*) is now quite common.

The practice of combining drugs to treat rheumatoid arthritis is analogous to how doctors manage other chronic conditions such as hypertension (high blood pressure). If one drug gives partial control, it is usually not stopped in favor of another drug, but rather a second drug is prescribed. Sometimes a third, fourth and or even fifth drug may be added. With many available options, it is possible to aim for complete control of blood pressure. Similarly, it is possible to aim for complete control of inflammation in rheumatoid arthritis using as many drugs as might be necessary and safe.

WHAT SHOULD YOU WORRY ABOUT WHEN TAKING METHOTREXATE?

A number of warnings are often given to patients concerning the use of methotrexate, which can often seem very distressing. It is important to be familiar with the possible side effects of methotrexate, but it is also important to recognize that most of these are quite unusual.

- **Methotrexate can reduce the formation of normal blood cells.** A check of blood cell counts is needed every four to eight weeks. However, with low-dose methotrexate, decreases in blood counts are quite unusual, particularly when folic acid is used as a supplement.
- **Methotrexate is a liver toxin.** Some doctors will suggest complete abstinence from alcohol, although other doctors consider it reasonable to suggest that a person could have one or two alcoholic drinks per day. All doctors agree that heavy use of alcohol is very dangerous while taking methotrexate. Patients using methotrexate should be given liver blood tests every four to six weeks to monitor the effect of the drug on the liver.
- **Methotrexate can cause a form of pneumonia.** This association is generally not suspected because we usually associate pneumonia with a bacterium or other type of infection, rather than with a chemical, such as a drug used to treat arthritis. So it is impor-

tant for anyone who takes methotrexate to be aware of this possible effect. After the pneumonia is better, most people can take methotrexate again a few weeks later without any problem. This finding has been interpreted to suggest that there may be an infection, as well as methotrexate, causing the pneumonia. Nonetheless, the pneumonia gets better when methotrexate is stopped. The pneumonia associated with methotrexate is the most feared side effect in people who take the drug for rheumatoid arthritis at this time.

• **Methotrexate can cause changes in the genetic structure of cells.** Such a genetic change theoretically may make a person vulnerable to development of cancer. However, this is a most unlikely event when low-dose methotrexate is used for rheumatoid arthritis. Many studies have shown that any possible increased risk of cancer in methotrexate-treated patients is minimal.

• **Methotrexate is teratogenic.** This means that it can lead to a risk of abnormalities in the development of a baby if a woman becomes pregnant while taking methotrexate. Women of childbearing years who are not exercising birth control should not use methotrexate. Also, men should not take this drug if the couple is trying to conceive.

• **Methotrexate can cause hair loss.** This problem can often be controlled by reducing the dose of methotrexate. Sometimes discontinuation is necessary.

• **Methotrexate can cause mouth sores.** Mouth sores or oral ulcers are common with methotrexate. Again, this problem can be reduced by lowering the dosage, giving folic acid along with the methotrexate, and/or with mouthwash treatment.

Despite the list of side effects with methotrexate treatment, it may help to remember that more than 60 percent of people who start methotrexate take it for longer than five years, and more than 40 percent take it longer than 10 years. Low-dose methotrexate can be thought of as a real milestone in the development of an effective treatment for rheumatoid arthritis.

Other Disease-Modifying Antirheumatic Drugs (DMARDs)

Although methotrexate is the most widely used DMARD, and many people are now taking some of the newer immune-response modulating drugs, there is still a place in treatment for traditional DMARDs. These include hydroxychloroquine, sulfasalazine, injectable gold, penicillamine and azathioprine, which may be used in combination with methotrexate or another DMARD. We will also briefly discuss cyclophosphamide, which, strictly-speaking, is not a DMARD, but is used to treat potentially life-threatening forms of rheumatoid arthritis such as rheumatoid vasculitis.

HYDROXYCHLOROQUINE

Hydroxychloroquine (*Plaquenil*) is an antimalarial drug that is of great benefit to some people with rheumatoid arthritis. This discovery was originally made with a related compound known as chloroquine (*Aralen*). Chloroquine was given to travelers to prevent malaria. Some travelers who took chloroquine also had rheumatoid arthritis, and reported dramatic benefit for their rheumatoid arthritis. Controlled clinical trials of antimalarial drugs for rheumatoid arthritis showed substantial benefit compared to placebo (or inert element).

A major barrier to the use of chloroquine was that it caused vision to be impaired in a very small number of patients. It certainly sounds scary to hear about eye complications, but fortunately these are relatively rare and can be detected early and addressed if you get regular eye exams.

Hydroxychloroquine is derived from chloroquine and has a much lower incidence of side effects related to the eye. In fact, one can calculate that the likelihood of serious eye toxicity with hydroxychloroquine is much lower than the likelihood of a person being involved in a motor vehicle accident. This does not mean that these events do not occur, but they should not be a major concern for people with rheumatoid arthritis. However, people taking hydroxychloroquine should have an eye exam at least every year or two.

In general, antimalarial drugs are very well tolerated. There are sometimes gastrointestinal distress and rash, as is the case with almost all drugs. There are no problems with blood tests or liver or kidney function associated with the use of antimalarial drugs.

SULFASALAZINE

Sulfasalazine (*Azulfidine*) was synthesized with a goal of treating rheumatoid arthritis. It is composed of two molecular components: one is a sulfa molecule such as found in antibiotics, and the other is a salicylate molecule such as is found in aspirin. Sulfasalazine is far superior to a placebo (or inert element) in clinical trials.

An important barrier to the use of sulfasalazine is gastrointestinal distress. Most people with rheumatoid arthritis tolerate 1-2 grams per day very well, but many people have distress even when doses are raised to 2-4 grams per day. Sulfasalazine is often used in combinations. In fact, the combination of methotrexate, hydroxychloroquine and sulfasalazine has been found to be substantially more effective than methotrexate alone in people who have incomplete response to methotrexate.

INJECTABLE GOLD

Gold injections were the most widely used treatment for rheumatoid arthritis from the 1950s through the 1980s, and continue to be widely used in certain centers. Gold was first used early in the 20th century because it was thought that rheumatoid arthritis might be caused by an infection (see Chapter 2), and gold was recognized to be a somewhat effective treatment for infections before antibiotics were developed. During the 1930s, a French rheumatologist named Forrestier began to use gold injections systematically. His work led to the establishment of injectable gold as the major treatment for rheumatoid arthritis from the 1940s to the 1980s.

Although injections of gold were associated with substantial improvement in about two-thirds of patients, side effects were common. The side effects included rash, kidney problems, blood cell abnormalities and lung problems, requiring discontinuation within a few months in more than one-third of patients. Perhaps as important was that many people who experienced a good response over three months to a year lost this response over time. Within two years, only about one-quarter of people who had begun gold treatment continued it.

Injectable gold is usually given as a 10-mg test dose of *Myochrysine* or *Solganol*, two different preparations of gold, followed by a 25-mg dose and then a 50-mg dose at weekly intervals. If the 50-mg dose is well tolerated, the patient is treated with 50-mg injections every week for 20 weeks. The injections are then given every two weeks, three weeks or even four weeks on a relatively indefinite basis, as long as the treatment appears effective and well tolerated – even if additional medications appear necessary. One problem in the use of gold is that its onset of action is relatively slow – it may take up to three months or sometimes longer to see an effect.

Even after five years, about 10 to 20 percent of people who take gold injections continue to have a good response. The combination of gold with methotrexate

has been studied, particularly in Europe, where results suggest it is a valuable combination for certain people.

ORAL GOLD

Oral gold or auranofin (*Ridaura*) was developed in the 1980s as a potential substitute for injectable gold. In clinical trials, it was found to be as effective as injectable gold, but these trials generally involved people with rheumatoid arthritis who had not taken other DMARDs previously and did not have longstanding disease. Oral gold is still used in people with *early* rheumatoid arthritis, but in long-term cases it does not seem as effective as many other drugs. The side effects are similar to injectable gold, but oral gold is better tolerated. It is sometimes used in combination with methotrexate or other DMARDs.

PENICILLAMINE

Penicillamine (*Depen* or *Cuprimine*) was first used in rheumatoid arthritis because it binds rheumatoid factor, although how it does this is still unclear. Penicillamine is a little like gold in that it is associated with occasional dramatic responses, but only about 10 percent to 20 percent have satisfactory long-term responses. Most doctors use a "go low, go slow" approach, beginning with 250 mg for a few weeks, increasing by 250 mg every four to eight weeks, up to 1,000 or even 1,500 mg per day as needed.

Although penicillamine leads to dramatic results in a few patients, use of penicillamine, like gold, is limited by side effects in 30 percent to 50 percent of patients who take it for less than six months. These side effects include rash, inflammation of the kidneys, effects on production of blood cells, gastrointestinal distress and, in a few people, a peculiar autoimmune syndrome that resembles lupus (see Chapter 3).

Penicillamine has been tried in several combinations but it is not used often in the modern treatment of rheumatoid arthritis.

AZATHIOPRINE

Azathioprine (*Imuran*) was the first immunosuppressive drug approved for use in rheumatoid arthritis. It controls the production of cells that account for inflammation. At this time, azathioprine is used most of the time as a supplement to methotrexate or in people who cannot tolerate methotrexate because of the side effects.

Azathioprine does not appear to be as effective as methotrexate, which hypothetically has a similar mechanism of action. Patients who take azathioprine require monitoring every four to eight weeks for blood counts and potential side effects on the liver. Azathioprine has been used in combination with methotrexate, and a few people showed significant improvement. In most people with rheumatoid arthritis, however, there was no major additional benefit from azathioprine.

CYCLOPHOSPHAMIDE

Cyclophosphamide (*Cytoxan*) is another immunosuppressive drug that was used by some rheumatologists in the 1970s in people with severe rheumatoid arthritis. It was effective in many people, but carried a high likelihood of severe side effects, including a risk of sterility, bladder complications and a higher risk of cancer. Cyclophosphamide is a potent *cytotoxic* agent that leads to profound suppression of the immune system, but it is not used except in life-threatening situations, such as a vasculitis that threatens to damage or destroy the heart or kidneys. Therefore, cyclophosphamide is no longer used to treat rheumatoid arthritis.

MINOCYCLINE

Minocycline (*Minocin*), though technically an antibiotic and not a DMARD, is a drug sometimes prescribed for treating rheumatoid arthritis. It is not yet approved by the FDA for this particular use. Side effects of minocycline include dizziness, vaginal infections, nausea, headache and skin rash. People who are sensitive to tetracycline medications may not want to use minocycline.

Immunomodulating Drugs

Four drugs that have become available for rheumatoid arthritis over the last five years represent a new generation of treatment. These drugs are able to target specific abnormal functions of the immune system directly. They include cyclosporine, leflunomide, etanercept and infliximab. Each of these drugs has a somewhat different mechanism of action and is taken in a different way.

CYCLOSPORINE

Cyclosporine (*Neoral*) was originally developed to prevent organ rejection in people who received organ transplants. It reduces the immune response through regulatory T cells (see Chapter 2), which are directly affected by the drug. Cyclosporine can be effective as a single drug for people with rheumatoid arthritis, and has been demonstrated to be effective when used in combination with methotrexate.

The dosage of cyclosporine is customized for each patient to get the best benefit and least likelihood of side effects. The starting dosage may be increased if there are no side effects on blood pressure and kidney function, and can be decreased if these side effects are seen, or when there is excellent control of disease.

The side effects of cyclosporine include upset stomach, nausea, loss of appetite and increased hair growth. The most severe complication of cyclosporine is its effect on the kidneys. Blood pressure, which is regulated by the kidneys, may become elevated and kidney function may be compromised. Your kidney function is monitored carefully with a blood test and measurement of blood pressure taken every two weeks at first, and every month or two thereafter. There is also a suggestion of some increased risk of cancer with long-term use of cyclosporine.

LEFLUNOMIDE

Leflunomide (*Arava*) is another compound that affects the immune response directly by blocking metabolic pathways important to the immune system. It is quite effective for people with rheumatoid arthritis, both as a single agent and in combination with methotrexate. Unlike cyclosporine, the dose of leflunomide is generally the same for each person. The typical dose is 100 mg for three days (a loading dose), and then 20 mg per day thereafter. Side effects include rashes and gastrointestinal symptoms but primarily, effects on liver function. In theory, this would make combination with methotrexate unlikely because methotrexate also can harm the liver. Research studies, however, have shown that methotrexate and leflunomide can be combined safely.

ETANERCEPT

Etanercept (*Enbrel*) is an entirely new kind of drug specifically designed to treat rheumatoid arthritis. Etanercept blocks a major component of inflammation known as tumor necrosis factor (TNF). This factor is critical in the inflammatory response. Etanercept blocks the action of TNF to help reduce inflammation. Some people have very dramatic responses to this drug.

Etanercept is given twice per week as an injection under the skin. In most cases, patients inject themselves, but some have a relative, friend or nurse do the injection. Side effects are minimal in that etanercept is well tolerated and doesn't interfere with blood counts. There is occasional local irritation at the site of injection. There is also a concern that because it may block the inflammatory response too effectively, etanercept may make it harder for the body to fight infection. Therefore, it is recommended that etanercept not be started if a severe infection is present, and the drug withheld should the patient develop an infection. In addition, possible long-term effects are unknown. Theoretically, a person may be more susceptible to cancer after taking this drug, but no evidence has emerged thus far that this is the case. Indeed, there were similar concerns about methotrexate 15 years ago, but they have not proven to be a real problem.

One other drawback of etanercept is that it is quite expensive. Insurance companies and managed-care organizations may be resistant to its use unless the disease was not controlled with another DMARD, because it may cost at least 10 times as much as most of the other medications for rheumatoid arthritis – as much as $1,200 per month. Nonetheless, etanercept is an excellent drug to try because total remission may be attained, something not often possible with other drugs.

INFLIXIMAB

Like etanercept, infliximab (*Remicade*) is designed to block the action of tumor necrosis factor (TNF) in the body. At this time, infliximab is only approved by the FDA for use in combination with methotrexate.

Infliximab is also given as an injection but in a very different way from etanercept.

Patients receive an intravenous infusion once every one to two months in a doctor's office, specialized clinic or hospital. The side effects of infliximab are also relatively few, although the same concerns regarding infection, as with etanercept, are present. It is possible that this drug, like etanercept, may be withheld in the face of active infection. Infliximab is also very expensive, with an annual cost in the same range as etanercept.

This new generation of drugs appears to take the treatment of rheumatoid arthritis to a new level not seen previously. Infliximab and etanercept have been used in combination with methotrexate, and many people appear to receive additional benefit by combining these drugs.

Combination Therapy

It is now clear that no single drug is likely to be a magic bullet to alleviate all the inflammation and pain associated with rheumatoid arthritis. Many different types of inflammatory chemicals and abnormalities of the inflammatory response are seen, and it would not be unreasonable to imagine that at least a few different drugs may be required to control the disease process. Because each DMARD works by a different mechanism of action, it might be expected that combining them would add to controlling inflammation and preventing damage.

Research studies have shown that combining certain DMARDs adds considerable benefit without any need to monitor the combination more than a single DMARD, and with no higher likelihood of side effects. As always, it is important to let your doctor know about any medications you are taking for conditions other than your arthritis.

By now you no doubt recognize that there is no single best drug for all people with rheumatoid arthritis. Each individual is unique, and each of the drugs available for this disease will work better for some people than others. There certainly are some drugs that a much larger proportion of the population will find helpful – such as low-dose prednisone and low-dose methotrexate – but you may find one of the other available drugs best for your own case. Because many people will be treated by combining different drugs, it is important to recognize that certain combinations will be better for some people, and other combinations better for others with rheumatoid arthritis.

Prosorba Column

In addition to drugs, another treatment for rheumatoid arthritis that should be noted here is protein A immunoadsorption therapy. In this therapy, patients have a needle, and then a catheter, placed in each arm. Blood is drawn from one arm, and run through a machine that separates plasma from red blood cells, known as an apheresis machine. The plasma is filtered through a *Prosorba column* to remove antibodies and immune complexes that promote inflammation. The plasma is joined again with the red blood cells, then infused through a

catheter into the other arm. The procedure is repeated weekly for 12 weeks.

Side-effects of this treatment include chills, flu-like symptoms, nausea or vomiting during the procedure and for several hours afterward. Rheumatoid arthritis may flare briefly after a procedure, but will stabilize. In the best cases, the rheumatoid arthritis will subside for 12 to 18 months.

Research and Development: Hope for the Future

There are several promising new drugs and therapies to treat rheumatoid arthritis currently in development and under study. Some of the drugs discussed in this chapter have become available recently, and already are being prescribed for many people with rheumatoid arthritis.

You may hear news about pharmaceutical companies conducting research on treating rheumatoid arthritis, and trying to develop new drugs. Be aware that the process takes time – approval by the federal government's Food and Drug Administration (FDA) for a new drug is the result of years of thorough testing to make sure the drug is safe and effective.

A number of new drugs designed to treat rheumatoid arthritis are in the FDA's approval process now. Many treatments are in the earliest stages of research and development at various pharmaceutical laboratories around the world. It is an exciting time for the development of rheumatoid arthritis drugs, with many new treatments likely to be approved in the next few years.

Remember that "new" does not always mean "better," especially if you are doing well with your current treatment. But the outlook for people with rheumatoid arthritis has never been better at any time in history. Research on new drugs to treat rheumatoid arthritis is active and ongoing.

You may learn about new or potential drugs on the news, or read reports on the Internet. When you hear that a drug has just been approved by the FDA, you may wish to ask your doctor or other health professional for more information to find out if it is a potential treatment for you.

Drugs Used in Treating Rheumatoid Arthritis

NSAIDS: NONSTEROIDAL ANTI-INFLAMMATORY DRUGS

Note: Possible side effects for all NSAIDs, except where noted, include abdominal pain, dizziness, drowsiness, fluid retention, gastric ulcers and bleeding, greater susceptibility to bruising or bleeding from cuts, heartburn, indigestion, lightheadedness, nausea, nightmares, rash, ringing in the ears, reduction in kidney function, increase in liver enzymes.

Ulcers or internal bleeding can occur without warning, so regular checkups are important. If you consume more than three alcoholic drinks per day, check with your doctor before using these products.

Aspirin
Brand names: *Anacin, Ascriptin, Bayer, Bufferin, Ecotrin, Excedrin Tablets, ZORprin, others*
Dosage: 3,600 to 5,400 mg per day in several doses

Choline magnesium trisalicylate
Brand names: *CMT, Tricosal, Trilisate*
Dosage: 3,000 mg per day in 2 or 3 doses
Other possible side effects: Bloating, confusion, deafness, diarrhea

Choline salicylate
Brand name: *Arthropan*
Dosage: 3,480 to 6,960 mg per day in several doses
Other possible side effects: Bloating, confusion, deafness, diarrhea

Diclofenac potassium
Brand name: *Cataflam*
Dosage: 100 to 200 mg per day in 3 or 4 doses

Diclofenac sodium
Brand name: *Voltaren*
Dosage: 150 to 200 mg per day in 3 or 4 doses

Diflunisal
Brand name: *Dolobid*
Dosage: 500 to 1,500 mg per day in 2 or 3 doses

Etodolac
Brand names: *Lodine, Lodine XL*
Dosage: 600 to 1,200 mg per day in 3 or 4 doses for *Lodine;* 400 to 1,000 mg per day in a single dose for *Lodine XL*

Drugs Used in Treating Rheumatoid Arthritis (cont.)

Fenoprofen calcium
Brand name: *Nalfon*
Dosage: 900 to 2,400 per day in 3 or 4 doses; never more than 3,200 mg per day

Flurbiprofen
Brand name: *Ansaid*
Dosage: 200 to 300 mg per day in 2 to 4 doses

Ibuprofen
Brand names: *Advil, Motrin, Motrin IB, Mediprin, Nuprin*
Dosage: 1,200 to 3,200 mg per day in 3 or 4 doses for prescription-strength *Motrin*; 200 to 400 mg every 4 to 6 hours as needed, not exceeding 1,200 mg per day, for over-the-counter brands

Indomethacin
Brand name: *Indocin, Indocin SR*
Dosage: 50 to 200 mg per day in 2 to 4 doses for *Indocin*; 75 mg per day in 1 dose, or 150 mg per day in 2 doses for *Indocin SR*.
Other possible side effects: Depression, headache, "spacey" feeling

Ketoprofen
Brand names: *Actron, Orudis, Orudis-KT, Oruvail*
Dosage: 200 to 225 mg per day in 3 or 4 doses for *Orudis*; 200 mg per day in a single dose for *Oruvail*; 12.5 mg every 4 to 6 hours as needed for *Actron* and *Orudis-KT*

Magnesium salicylate
Brand names: *Magan, Doan's Pills, Mobidin, Arthritab*
Dosage: 2,600 to 4,800 mg per day in 3 to 6 doses
Other possible side effects: Bloating, confusion, deafness, diarrhea

Meclofenamate sodium
Brand name: *Meclomen*
Dosage: 200 to 400 mg per day in 4 doses

Mefenamic acid
Brand name: *Ponstel*
Dosage: 1,000 mg per day in 4 doses

Meloxicam
Brand name: *Mobic*
Dosage: No approved dosage for RA; ask your physician

Nabumetone
Brand name: *Relafen*
Dosage: 500 to 1,000 mg per day in 1 or 2 doses

Naproxen
Brand names: *Naprosyn, Naprelan*
Dosage: 500 to 1,500 mg per day in 2 doses for *Naprosyn;* 750 or 1,000 mg per day in a single dose for *Naprelan*

Naproxen sodium
Brand names: *Anaprox, Aleve*
Dosage: 550 to 1,100 mg per day in 2 doses for *Anaprox;* 220 mg every 8 to 12 hours as needed for *Aleve*

Oxaprozin
Brand name: *Daypro*
Dosage: 1,200 mg per day in a single dose or 1,800 mg per day in 2 doses

Piroxicam
Brand name: *Feldene*
Dosage: 20 mg per day in 1 or 2 doses

Salsalate
Brand names: *Disalcid, Mono-gesic, Salflex, Salsitab, Arnigesic, Anaflex 750, Marthritic*
Dosage: 1,000 to 3,000 mg per day in 2 or 3 doses
Other possible side effects: Bloating, confusion, deafness, diarrhea

Sodium salicylate
Brand name: None, generic only
Dosage: 3,600 to 5,400 mg per day in several doses
Other possible side effects: Bloating, confusion, deafness, diarrhea

Sulindac
Brand name: *Clinoril*
Dosage: 300 to 400 mg per day in 2 doses

Tolmetin sodium
Brand name: *Tolectin*
Dosage: 1,200 mg per day in 3 doses

Drugs Used in Treating Rheumatoid Arthritis (cont.)

COX-2 INHIBITORS

Note: This new class of NSAIDs blocks the prostaglandins involved in inflammation, but not the prostaglandins that protect the stomach lining. Therefore, COX-2 inhibitors may not have the stomach-related side effects of traditional NSAIDs. They also may not provide the same protection against heart attacks and strokes.

Celecoxib
Brand name: *Celebrex*
Dosage: 200 to 400 mg per day in 2 doses
Possible side effects: Same as other NSAIDs, except less likely to cause gastric ulcers and susceptibility to bruising and bleeding

Rofecoxib
Brand name: *Vioxx*
Dosage: Indication not sought for rheumatoid arthritis; ask your physician
Possible side effects: Same as other NSAIDs, except less likely to cause gastric ulcers and susceptibility to bruising and bleeding

ANALGESICS

These are drugs used for pain relief. Other than acetaminophen, these drugs have the potential for dependence if used for long periods of time.

Acetaminophen
Brand names: *Anacin (aspirin-free), Excedrin caplets, Panadol, Tylenol*
Dosage: 325 to 1,000 mg every 4 to 6 hours as needed; no more than 4,000 mg per day
Possible side effects: When taken as prescribed, acetaminophen is usually not associated with side effects

Acetaminophen with codeine
Brand names: *Fioricet, Phenaphen with codeine, Tylenol with codeine*
Dosage: 15 to 60 mg every 4 hours as needed
Possible side effects: Constipation, dizziness or lightheadedness, drowsiness, nausea, unusual tiredness or weakness, vomiting

Propoxyphene hydrochloride
Brand names: *Darvon, PC-Cap, Wygesic*
Dosage: 65 mg every 4 hours as needed; no more than 390 mg per day
Possible side effects: Dizziness or lightheadedness, drowsiness, nausea and vomiting

Tramadol
Brand name: *Ultram*
Dosage: 50 to 100 mg every 6 hours as needed
Possible side effects: Dizziness, nausea, constipation, headache, sleepiness

GLUCOCORTICOIDS

Note: Side effects may be minimal when glucocorticoids are taken short-term or at very low doses. The following side effects are possible for all the following glucocorticoids, but are more common with high doses and long-term use: Cushing's syndrome (weight gain, moon-face, thin skin, muscle weakness, brittle bones), cataracts, hypertension, increased appetite, elevated blood sugar, indigestion, insomnia, mood changes, nervousness or restlessness.

Dosage varies greatly based on disease severity.

Cortisone
Brand names: *Cortone Acetate*
Dosage: 5 to 150 mg per day in a single dose

Dexamethasone
Brand names: *Decadron, Hexadrol*
Dosage: 0.5 to 9 mg per day in a single dose

Hydrocortisone
Brand names: *Cortef, Hydrocortone*
Dosage: 20 to 240 mg per day in a single dose or divided into several doses

Methylprednisolone
Brand name: *Medrol*
Dosage: 4 to 160 mg per day in a single dose or divided into several doses

Prednisolone
Brand name: *Prelone*
Dosage: 5 to 200 mg per day in a single dose or divided into several doses

Prednisolone sodium phosphate (liquid only)
Brand name: *Pediapred*
Dosage: 5 to 60 ml per day in 1 to 3 doses

Drugs Used in Treating Rheumatoid Arthritis (cont.)

Prednisone
Brand names: *Deltasone, Orasone, Prednicen-M, Sterapred*
Dosage: 1 to 60 mg per day in a single dose or divided into several doses

Triamcinolone
Brand name: *Aristocort*
Dosage: 4 to 60 mg per day in a single dose or divided into several doses

BIOLOGIC RESPONSE MODIFIERS

Note: This new class of arthritis drugs block TNF (tumor necrosis factor), believed to play a major role in causing inflammation and joint damage. They may make patients more susceptible to infections. Little is known about their long-term side effects.

Etanercept
Brand name: *Enbrel*
Dosage: 25 mg twice per week, given by subcutaneous (beneath the skin) injection
Possible side effects: Redness and/or itching, pain or swelling at the injection site

Infliximab
Brand name: *Remicade*
Dosage: Determined by body weight. Drug is infused intravenously in a two-hour outpatient procedure every 1 to 2 months. Only approved for use in combination with methotrexate in rheumatoid arthritis.
Possible side effects: Upper respiratory infection, headache, nausea, coughing

DMARDs – DISEASE-MODIFYING ANTIRHEUMATIC DRUGS – and Others

Note: Minocycline, an antibiotic, is included here, since it has been shown to be effective in treating rheumatoid arthritis. Many DMARDs are used in combination to increase effectiveness and decrease side effects. Comprehensive explanations of cautions are in this chapter.

Auranofin (oral gold)
Brand name: *Ridaura*
Dosage: 6 to 9 mg per day in 1 or 2 doses
Possible side effects: Abdominal or stomach cramps or pain, bloated feeling, decrease in or loss of appetite, diarrhea or loose stools, gas or indigestion, mouth sores, nausea or vomiting, skin rash or itching

Azathioprine
Brand name: *Imuran*
Dosage: 50 to 150 mg per day in 1 to 3 doses, based on body weight
Possible side effects: Cough, fever and chills, loss of appetite, nausea or vomiting, skin rash, unusual bleeding or bruising, unusual tiredness or weakness

Cyclophosphamide
Brand name: *Cytoxan*
Dosage: 50 to 150 mg per day in a single dose; may also be given intravenously
Possible side effects: Blood in urine or burning on urination, confusion or agitation, cough, dizziness, fever and chills, infertility in men and women, loss of appetite, missed menstrual periods, nausea or vomiting, unusual bleeding or bruising, unusual tiredness or weakness

Cyclosporine
Brand names: *Sandimmune, Neoral*
Dosage: 100 to 400 mg per day in 2 doses; dose is based on body weight
Possible side effects: Tender or enlarged gums, high blood pressure, increase in hair growth, kidney problems, loss of appetite, tremors

Injectable gold
Brand names: Gold sodium thiolomate: *Myochrysine;* Aurothioglucose: *Solganol*
Dosage: 10 mg in a single dose the first week, 25 mg the following week, then 25 to 50 mg per week thereafter. Frequency may be reduced after several months.
Possible side effects: Irritation or soreness or tongue, metallic taste, skin rash or itching, soreness, swelling or bleeding of gums, unusual bleeding or bruising

Hydroxychloroquine sulfate
Brand name: *Plaquenil*
Dosage: 200 to 600 mg per day in 1 or 2 doses
Possible side effects: Black spots in visual field, diarrhea, loss of appetite, nausea, rash

Leflunomide
Brand name: *Arava*
Dosage: 10 to 20 mg per day in a single dose
Possible side effects: Diarrhea, skin rash, liver toxicity, hair loss

Drugs Used in Treating Rheumatoid Arthritis (cont.)

Methotrexate
Brand name: *Rheumatrex*
Dosage: 7.5 to 25 mg per week in 3 doses, or 10 mg per week in a single dose; may also be given by injection
Possible side effects: Cough, diarrhea, hair loss, loss of appetite, unusual bleeding or bruising, liver toxicity, lung toxicity

Minocycline
Brand name: *Minocin*
Dosage: 200 mg per day in 2 doses
Possible side effects: Dizziness, vaginal infections, nausea, headache, skin rash

Penicillamine
Brand names: *Cuprimine, Depen*
Dosage: 125 to 250 mg per day in a single dose to start, increased to not more than 1,500 mg per day in 3 doses
Possible side effects: Diarrhea, joint pain, lessening or loss of sense of taste, loss of appetite, fever, hives or itching, mouth sores, nausea or vomiting, skin rash, stomach pain, swollen glands, unusual bleeding or bruising, weakness

Sulfasalazine
Brand name: *Azulfidine*
Dosage: 2 to 3 grams per day in 2 to 4 doses
Possible side effects: Stomach upset, diarrhea, dizziness, headache, light sensitivity, itching, appetite loss, liver abnormalities, lowered blood count, nausea or vomiting, rash

For more arthritis drug information, *Arthritis Today* publishes an annual Drug Guide that is available free of charge by calling 800/283-7800, or on the Arthritis Foundation Web site, www.arthritis.org.

Chapter 12

Surgery:

Opening New Doors

For many people with rheumatoid arthritis, surgery is an important treatment option at certain points in their disease, used in addition to elements of treatment like medication, exercise, physical and occupational therapy, and joint protection.

Many surgical procedures for people with arthritis are now available, and they can contribute greatly to relieving pain and improving function. The development of these surgical options over the last 35 years certainly must be included as one of the major breakthroughs in helping people with arthritis remain active and continue to enjoy life.

Joint surgery may be performed early or late in the disease course, depending on the procedure. For example, in early disease a synovectomy (the surgical removal of the *synovium*, or lining of the joint) may be performed when one or two specific joints are affected by inflammation much more than most other joints. In later disease, an *arthrodesis* or fusion of a joint may greatly relieve pain. After a joint is severely damaged, a total joint replacement (most commonly of a hip or knee) may dramatically relieve pain and improve a person's ability to function.

In this chapter, we will discuss the types of surgery that may be helpful to people with rheumatoid arthritis. In addition, we will present guidelines regarding what to expect from surgery, remembering as always that each person is different. Information will be provided about what you can do – both before and after the operation – to increase the chances of success.

Common Surgical Procedures

SYNOVECTOMY

The *synovium* is the protective lining of the joint. When one or two joints, such as a wrist or knee, stands out as much more severely involved than other joints, a synovectomy may be performed. This procedure is designed to remove diseased synovium, and will reduce the amount of inflammatory tissue, which will relieve swelling and pain. As a result, damage to the joint may be slowed or even prevented. However, the synovium may grow back after several years, and the problem may recur.

Synovectomies are usually performed in the wrist, elbow or knee, and they may be combined with resection (see below). If the inflammation has caused tendons to rupture, then repair and reconstruction of these tendons may be done simultaneously to improve function. Tendon rupture is rather unusual except in people with rheumatoid arthritis or cases of injury.

ARTHROSCOPIC SURGERY

An *arthroscope* is an instrument that consists of a very thin tube with a light at the end that is inserted into the joint through a small incision. Arthroscopic surgery has become more and more common over the last 20 years because it involves smaller incisions than traditional surgery, leading to a quicker recovery in most people. In addition, certain types of repairs can be done more easily through an arthroscope.

Arthroscopy can be used to view the inside of a joint. The arthroscope is connected to a closed-circuit television, allowing the doctor to see inside the joint and estimate the extent of damage. The doctor then has many options, including taking samples of tissue for laboratory analysis, removing pieces of loose cartilage or other tissue that can cause pain, repairing a tear in the cartilage, smoothing a rough joint surface, or removing diseased synovial tissue, as a synovectomy (described above). Arthroscopic surgery can hypothetically be performed in virtually any joint, but is most commonly performed in the knee and shoulder.

OSTEOTOMY

The term *osteotomy* literally means "to cut bone." This procedure was used often in the past when joints were *malaligned,* or did not line up correctly as a result of damage to supporting structures and bone. The goal of the osteotomy was to increase stability by redistributing the weight on the joint. This was usually done in the hip or knee to shift the load of bearing weight from areas where the cartilage was damaged to areas that still had cartilage to cushion the load.

The procedure is still performed occasionally by cutting the bones whose ends do not line up properly and repositioning them to improve alignment. Osteotomy is generally performed to support weight bearing in the joints of the legs. Because of better control of inflammation, leading to fewer problems with alignment of joints, and improvements in the results of joint replacement surgery, osteotomies are relatively unusual in the treatment of rheumatoid arthritis at this time. In general, osteotomies are most successful in younger active people who have a good range of motion in the joint, good muscle function and some remaining cartilage around the joint.

RESECTION

Resection is a procedure that involves removing all or part of a bone. It was most commonly used years ago to relieve pain and improve function in the hands and wrists in early rheumatoid arthritis, and to protect the tendons from damage. It was often combined with synovectomy. Resection of damaged joints in the feet is still commonly performed to remove *bunions* in the large toe or *hammer toes* in the other toes. Resection can make walking less painful by removing parts of a bone that cause pressure.

Resection is sometimes used in conjunction with joint replacement – a procedure known as *resection arthroplasty*. This type of surgery is rarely used as a primary procedure today, however, due to the development of more successful types of joint replacement surgery. Resection procedures are only used commonly in the feet.

JOINT REPLACEMENT SURGERY

Of all the types of surgery available for people with arthritis, this is the one you've most likely heard about before. That's because joint replacement surgery is one of the biggest success stories in the treatment of chronic joint diseases like rheumatoid arthritis. Joint replacement surgery – or *arthroplasty* – is the surgical reconstruction or replacement of a joint. Joint replacement is available for different joints, most commonly the hip or knee. Joint replacement surgery has been extremely successful in enabling people who might previously have needed to use a wheelchair at times. Joint replacement is recommended most often for people older than age 50, but people whose rheumatoid arthritis developed in childhood or at an early age may require joint reconstruction sooner.

The procedure itself involves removing the damaged joint, resurfacing and relining the ends of bones where cartilage has worn away, and replacing the joint with one of several types of man-made components. The components used are made of metal, ceramic or plastic parts.

There are two different categories of replacement joints currently being used: cemented or cementless. Cemented joints are secured in place during surgery with a special cementing material called methylmethacrylate. Cementless joints usually have a porous surface that is fitted next to the bone. Over time, the bone will grow into the joint and hold it in place without

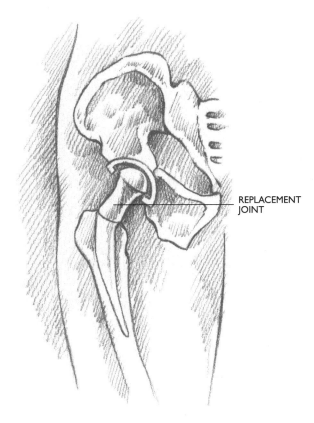

REPLACEMENT JOINT

HIP REPLACEMENT

the need for cement. In general, cement-less replacements are thought to last longer than cemented joints in most, but not all, people. In addition, they usually lead to better bone *remodeling* (the regrowth of bone around the prosthetic joint) and easier *revision* (replacing the artificial joint), if necessary. However, uncemented joint replacements usually require a longer peri-od of limited weight bearing (such as using crutches or a cane) after surgery. The deci-sion about a cemented or cementless joint replacement varies from one person to another.

Unfortunately, joint replacements may not last forever. The cement may loosen over time, or one of the components may break. In the early days of joint replacement surgery, about 30 years ago, the replaced joint might have been expected to last only five to 10 years or so. But improvements in both artifi-cial joints and surgical techniques have expanded the life span to 15 years or more. Many people can anticipate that a joint replaced at this time may last indefinitely. If the joint replacement breaks down over time, revision arthroplasty is often very successful, and further replacement is not needed.

ARTHRODESIS (FUSION)

Arthrodesis is a surgical procedure that fuses two bones together. Although arthrode-sis will limit movement, it is usually done to relieve pain and to increase stability in the ankles, wrists, fingers and toes. It may also be performed in the spine, fusing two or more

vertebrae together to stabilize the spine and eliminate pain. Occasionally, when joint replacement surgery is unsuccessful, the site becomes infected or surrounding structures are extensively destroyed, arthrodesis of the hip or knee provides another surgical option.

In arthrodesis, the bones forming a joint are joined together, often using bones from the patient's pelvis – or sometimes metallic or plastic hardware – to hold the bones in place until they begin to grow and fuse together. The resulting fused joint will lose flexibility, but will be less painful, more sta-ble and often more capable of functions such as pinching fingers or bearing weight.

What You Can Expect From Surgery

In most cases, surgery for people with rheumatoid arthritis is an elective procedure, which means that it is performed by choice and not because it is medically urgent or because of a potentially life-threatening situ-ation (such as the removal of an inflamed appendix to prevent rupture). Nevertheless, it is undeniably a medically important pro-cedure that may dramatically relieve pain and restore lost function and independence.

DECIDING ON SURGERY

Suppose your doctor has suggested that you may benefit from undergoing one of the surgical procedures discussed above. Most likely, you will have some time to consider your decision and discuss your options with your doctor and with the surgeon. Surgery may seem scary, but it is often the best treatment to help you lead a normal life.

Because elective joint replacement procedures are scheduled in advance, it is possible for you to find out quite a bit about the surgery ahead of time – including any risks that might be involved, how the procedure is done, the expected recovery time and how you can participate. As with all treatments, you should consider the risks as well as the benefits. Some of the risks associated with joint surgery include the following:

• **Anesthesia.** Certain risks are associated with the use of general anesthesia and should be discussed with your surgeon and *anesthesiologist* before the surgery.
• **Blood clots.** These can develop following surgery, particularly if the surgery is in your lower extremities. Blood clots are less common than they once were due to improvements in postoperative care.

• **Infection.** An infection can be introduced into the joint and can jeopardize the success of a joint replacement. In very rare instances, the infection may spread to other parts of your body through the bloodstream.
• **Weight.** Being overweight can slow recovery of a joint replacement in a weight-bearing joint by adding stress to it. Excess weight can also cause problems with the surgery itself, as it may make the procedure more difficult and a person more vulnerable to complications such as infection in the incision, lungs and other organs.

In addition to these general risks, a person with rheumatoid arthritis may encounter some particular problems with surgery. The drug program used to treat rheumatoid arthritis often must be adjusted prior to surgery, such as stopping NSAIDs and methotrexate for a week prior to surgery. Sometimes dosages can be lowered.

Personally Speaking   Stories from real people with rheumatoid arthritis

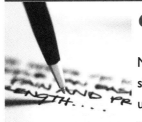

"We were visiting our daughter and her family in Michigan in our RV, and our grandchildren, ages 4 and 7, wanted to stay overnight with Nana and Grampa. The two children slept with Nana, and Grampa slept up front. During the night, my knee and hip began to hurt real bad. I reached for my rub in the darkness, so as not to wake up anyone. Well, I got my tube and proceeded to rub from knee to my hip. Boy, did I smell good! But I still hurt. Turning on the light, I realized that I had reached for the toothpaste.

That Minty-Fresh Feeling
by Barbara Reynolds, Holland Patent, NY

"My granddaughter will not let me forget my new arthritis rub!"

Checklist: Questions to Ask Before Surgery

1. Do I understand the procedure? Are there written materials, classes or videos of this surgery that I can review to help me understand?

2. Can I talk with someone who has experienced this procedure with this orthopaedic surgeon?

3. Will the surgery be done on an inpatient (a hospital stay) or outpatient basis? If I will be an inpatient, how long can I expect to be hospitalized after surgery?

4. What are the risks involved in this type of surgery? How likely are they to occur? Do I have any special risk factors?

5. What are the risks if I delay or choose not to have the surgery?

6. Is it likely that more surgery will be necessary?

7. What improvement can I expect from surgery? Is there any downside to this procedure (for example, loss of joint motion following arthrodesis)?

8. Will I need to stop taking any of my medications before surgery? How long before?

9. Can I arrange to have blood taken from me weeks before surgery so that if I need a blood transfusion because of blood loss during surgery, it can be my own blood (the safest form of transfusion)?

10. How much pain should I expect? How long will it last?

11. What exercise program is recommended before and after the operation?

12. When do I start physical therapy? Will it be in my home or at the therapist's office?

13. Will I need to arrange for assistance at home after the surgery? For how long?

14. Will I need any special equipment at home? Do I need to make any modifications in my home?

15. What limits will there be on my activities — driving, climbing stairs, returning to work, having sex — and for how long?

16. How often will I have follow-up visits? Will my rheumatologist be involved as well?

This must be carefully planned prior to surgery to avoid having a sudden flare of disease. Another consideration is the need for multiple surgeries. For instance, an individual may need to have surgery in the foot and ankle before planning to have a total knee replacement, so that rehabilitation will go well.

BEFORE SURGERY

Once you have decided to go ahead with surgery, you will need to make plans for the procedure. Your doctor's office will handle administrative details, such as getting pre-approvals for surgery. Many orthopaedic surgeons conduct educational programs concerning surgery, including classes, videos or individualized instruction. Take advantage of these programs – they can be very helpful.

The checklist on the previous page provides a list of questions that you may review, some of which you might think about during education programs and discuss with your doctor or other health professionals when you are preparing for surgery. Answers to these questions can guide you in making a decision to have surgery and in determining what to expect before, during and after the procedure.

AFTER THE SURGERY

As with any other component of your arthritis management plan, surgery – or rather, the recovery from surgery – requires your active participation for best results. The procedure itself is merely the first step in a longer process of rehabilitating the joint. The end result is worth the effort. Surgeries for arthritis effectively relieve pain and improve joint function.

There are many types of arthritis-related surgery, and some are more complicated than others, necessitating longer periods of recovery. For example, the rehabilitation required after knee replacement involves considerably more effort than that after hip replacement surgery, and the recovery from hip replacement is usually much more rapid.

In general, your surgeon and physical therapist will advise you to begin mobilizing your affected joint as soon as possible, sometimes even before your sutures heal. Movement should be gentle at first, gradually increasing as appropriate.

Within a few weeks of surgery, you should be able to get back to most of your daily activities. Following joint replacement surgery, recovery may take longer and certain activities may be prohibited for a period of several months. Every person is different; some people restrict their levels of certain activities following surgery according to their own needs. Returning to full-time activities is usually possible within three months of joint replacement.

A physical or occupational therapist usually is involved in the rehabilitation process. In some cases, a patient begins therapy in a hospital or postoperative rehabilitation facility, but many attend therapy sessions in an office setting. But only a small part of the rehabilitation is accomplished in a hospital, doctor's or therapist's office. Most of the exercise routine will be given to you to perform at home. It will be your goal to keep yourself motivated and to do your exercises faithfully and regularly. The payoff will be proportional to the amount of work you put into it.

Part Three

Managing Rheumatoid Arthritis:
What You Can Do

Chapter 13

Mind Power:

Getting Mentally Tough

Can rheumatoid arthritis really be affected by your outlook? The answer is yes. The major question is how much – and that probably differs greatly from person to person (like everything else with rheumatoid arthritis).

Exciting findings over the last few years indicate that how you react to the stresses and challenges of living with a chronic disease may have a direct influence on the course of the disease. Equally important, your outlook may influence your long-term ability to keep doing all the daily activities that make you independent and make your life meaningful.

There are many different strategies you can use to deal with your arthritis. Because every person is different, some of these techniques may work better for you than others. In this chapter, we will first discuss some ideas of how the mind-body connection works, and why it affects your arthritis. Then we will take a look at some of the techniques that have been shown to be effective self-management tools.

The Mind-Body Connection

In the past, doctors suggested there was something called the "rheumatoid arthritis personality." Some researchers had a theory that rheumatoid arthritis could be considered a *psychosomatic* disease – meaning that it was caused largely by "mental" processes that led to physical disease.

As we now know, this idea was a great oversimplification of a very complicated situation. There is no such thing as a rheumatoid arthritis personality; all types of people

get rheumatoid arthritis, and the disease affects different people in different ways. However, there was a germ of truth in the idea. It does appear that the mind plays some role in the disease process in rheumatoid arthritis – and in most diseases.

For instance, a person's reaction to stressful events probably has an effect on flares of rheumatoid arthritis in some, if not most, people. Continued stress appears to make it harder to control disease. There is evidence that people with optimistic outlooks and feelings of being in control tend to do better over the long-term than people with less positive feelings about their rheumatoid arthritis. This concept of being in control has become known as *self-efficacy*, and its opposite is known as *helplessness*. We'll discuss these cornerstones of mental strategies in this chapter.

Why Self-Efficacy Can Help

As you know, rheumatoid arthritis is a chronic, painful condition that can cause stress, frustration and depression, which in turn, make the pain worse. This cycle of pain is vicious, but it can be halted or reduced through treatment and by learning to deal with your pain in positive, constructive ways.

Some people who have rheumatoid arthritis may sometimes believe their situation is uncontrollable and there are no effective solutions to help them, a state of mind known as helplessness. These feelings may result in anxiety, depression and fear of the future. People may lose interest in daily living and cannot make the effort to learn new skills that could help them manage their pain and stress.

Self-efficacy, which refers to a person's feeling that she or he can master a specific situation, may help people with rheumatoid arthritis considerably. People who have good self-efficacy skills tend to be able to cope better with their disease than those who feel helpless in the face of their constantly fluctuating symptoms.

One important thing to remember about self-efficacy is that it is specific to situations, rather than an overall approach to coping

A Pioneer Course Still Going Strong

The **Arthritis Self-Management Program**, offered by the Arthritis Foundation as the Arthritis Self-Help Course, was first developed in 1979 by researchers Kate Lorig, RN, DrPH, and James Fries, MD. At that time, it was considered a groundbreaking idea to provide people with arthritis not only information about their disease but also skills to help them regain control of their lives. "The whole point of the course," explains Dr. Lorig, "is to help people have more confidence to manage their symptoms and be able to live a better life with their disease."

The program originally included information about exercises, muscle relaxation, joint protection, communication between doctors and patients, and taking medicines. As the course was revised over the years, Dr. Lorig found that the most important aspects were those that helped individuals develop their self-efficacy skills. These skills are now emphasized during the six-week program, along with cognitive pain management and aerobic exercises. The success of the course has spurred the development of other excellent programs that help people cope with chronic pain and learn self-efficacy techniques.

To locate an Arthritis Self-Help Course near you, check the Arthritis Foundation's Web site (www.arthritis.org) or call 800/283-7800 to find the Arthritis Foundation chapter nearest you. The chapter staff will be able to guide you to local resources in your area.

with pain and stress. Actually, a layman's term for self-efficacy is confidence. For instance, a person may have a high self-efficacy (or confidence level) for walking around the block but a low self-efficacy for climbing Mount Everest.

The good news is that helplessness may be overcome and self-efficacy skills can be learned. When researchers discovered the importance of optimism and self-efficacy, they began to develop programs and courses to help people with arthritis learn these valuable skills. One of the first of these programs – and still one of the most successful – is the Arthritis Self-Management Program, offered through the Arthritis Foundation as the Arthritis Self-Help Course (see p.118). During the six-week course, participants learn and practice self-efficacy skills that help them gain confidence in managing their disease.

Coping With Stress

Having rheumatoid arthritis increases your physical and emotional challenges. You may feel fear, anger and frustration about your pain or physical limitations. These emotions are normal, and are part of the process your body goes through to make sense of this new situation in your life. Some people are able to experience these emotions and simply move on, but many others who have rheumatoid arthritis find it difficult to deal with the ongoing stresses of chronic disease. Finding ways to reduce and handle stress should be an important component of your self-management plan.

WHAT IS STRESS?

Stress refers to the body's physical, mental and chemical reactions to frightening, exciting, dangerous or irritating circumstances. This can be anything from getting the children to school on time to avoiding a crash on the freeway. Every day we face hundreds of stresses – some big and some small – to which we must make appropriate responses.

When we face stress, our bodies are programmed to respond by releasing adrenaline, cortisol and other hormones into the bloodstream. These hormones increase your heart rate, blood pressure and muscle tension, and induce what has been called the "fight or flight response." This kind of response works just fine most of the time. The stress response can actually be beneficial, particularly during emergencies or in high-pressure situations. After a stressful situation is resolved, however, the body's pace needs to return to normal.

Unfortunately, stress levels in our modern society often remain high. You probably experience daily stress on the job, in traffic or because of your health. If you are unable to release tension between stressful situations, your body may start to respond to every pressure as if it's an emergency. Think of your body as a car: It's unhealthy to "race your engine" constantly. You need to shift into neutral sometimes to save wear and tear on your engine.

When the stress response continues for an extended period, it can wear you down. You may find yourself reaching overload and notice that you are accident-prone or that you are making more mistakes than usual. These are signs that you need to try to relieve some of the stress in your life.

MANAGING STRESS

By using methods that have been developed by clinicians and people with arthritis, and tested by researchers, you can learn to improve your own stress-management skills.

The first step is to identify what is causing stress in your life (these factors are called *stressors*). Second, you should try to eliminate as many stressors as possible. The third step is to develop effective coping mechanisms to help you counteract the stresses that you cannot eliminate. Some coping mechanisms that can help you manage stress include progressive muscle relaxation, guided imagery, deep breathing techniques and active problem solving.

Step one: Identifying stressors. Before you can change or manage your stress, you must become aware of what's causing it. Identifying your stressors is a process of personal discovery. Of course, there are universal stresses that affect every person's life, such as moving, changing jobs or having a baby. But other stressors are highly individual. What triggers stress for you may not necessarily bother someone else.

One way to discover what causes you stress is to keep a stress diary. The sample diary shown here is a way to note the things that cause you to feel "stressed out." Review your entries at the end of each week to see if there is a pattern of stress-related events. Some people find that this step alone can be empowering. Indeed, extensive research indicates that the simple act of writing down some of the difficulties can in itself lead to better outcomes.

The physical signs of stress can also provide clues and can be noted in your stress

Sample Stress Diary

DATE	CAUSE OF STRESS	TIME	PHYSICAL SYMPTOMS	EMOTIONAL SYMPTOMS
4/18	getting kids off to school	7 a.m.	fast heartbeat, tightness of neck	feel rushed, disorganized
4/18	stuck in traffic	8:30 a.m.	headache, heart beating faster, legs aching	frustrated, angry at being late
4/18	meeting presentation	10 a.m.	fast heartbeat, dry throat, clammy palms	anxious, nervous

diary as well. These include fatigue/exhaustion, tense muscles, upset stomach, insomnia, cold or sweaty hands, changes in appetite, teeth grinding, jaw clenching, and general body complaints such as weakness, dizziness, headache or muscle pain. You should be aware that many of these physical symptoms of stress are also symptoms of arthritis. For example, fatigue, weakness and muscle pain are common in rheumatoid arthritis, especially during a flare. Sometimes it's difficult to tell whether your symptoms are caused by stress or by disease – often it's both, or the same thing.

Your stress diary might also include emotional symptoms. These can range from

Stress Diary

Keep a diary or chart if you can and record the causes of your stress as well as physical or emotional symptoms you experience. Keeping a stress diary can help you learn what causes your stress and how you can avoid it.

DATE	CAUSE OF STRESS	TIME	PHYSICAL SYMPTOMS	EMOTIONAL SYMPTOMS

mild irritability to feelings of depression. Anxiety, nervousness and agitation are also common signs of stress. Try to be as specific as possible, so that you can target the most troublesome areas for you.

Step two: Eliminate the negative. Now comes the challenging part – trying to weed out negative pressures in your life. Obviously, not all negative stressors can be eliminated, and sometimes it's stressful just to think about making changes in your life. For instance, you may feel obligated to honor many family and volunteer duties. It may seem easier to continue doing them than to back out. People may pressure you not to change. But you need to realize that saying no to a few of these obligations may enable you to feel less stressed and have more energy for the things you really must do or want to do.

Review your stress diary. Are there predictable times during the day or week when you feel particularly hassled? For example, being stuck in rush-hour traffic may disrupt your equilibrium and deplete the energy you need to see you through the day. Brainstorm some options that could make your commute easier. Can you leave for work earlier? Can you carpool or take public transportation? Would listening to your favorite classical music make you feel more relaxed? Now try taking each problem you've identified and see if you can figure out ways to reduce the stress associated with each.

Carrying out this step may be especially difficult for people who pride themselves on their competency and efficiency. Try to remember that no one is immune to stressful stimuli. Try to adjust your mindset by

Putting Stress in Perspective

You can learn to take a more objective look at the stresses and stress-causing patterns in your life by asking yourself these questions:

- Does this situation reflect a threat that is signaling harm, or a challenge that is signaling an opportunity?
- Are there other ways to look at this situation?
- What exactly is at stake?
- What are you saying to yourself right now? Is it productive?
- What are you afraid will occur?
- What evidence do you have that this will happen?
- Is there evidence that contradicts this conclusion?
- What changes can you make?
- What coping resources are available to you?

remembering that the more stress you eliminate, the more productively you will be able to handle the tasks you must do. If you can take a step back and become more objective about your situation, it will be easier to evaluate and deal with stress (see box, p.122).

Step three: Develop effective coping mechanisms. A positive attitude can contribute to treating the cycle of stress in your life. This does not mean that simply looking on the sunny side of life can make a serious problem go away. Rather, it means that if you cultivate the ability to be flexible and learn how to deal with change, you will feel less stress and will be able to function more effectively in dealing with problems.

There are many ways to counteract stress positively. For example, if you find yourself dwelling on your problems, you can learn to refocus your attention on solving them and on positive things you enjoy. Thinking about something you like can help you relax and become less stressed. Also, humor is a wonderful way to relieve stress. Schedule time for play, and become involved in activities that make you laugh.

Another important key is to develop and use support systems. Sharing your thoughts with family, friends, clergy or other good listeners can help you view your problems in a constructive way. A support group of people who have arthritis may provide a valuable source of both listeners and information on dealing with stress.

When you feel that stress is about to overwhelm you, develop a "safety valve" proce-dure to let off steam. This could involve writing down your feelings in a journal, taking some time to calm down in a quiet setting, or exercising vigorously (but safely). Above all, try to keep a balance between your work, family and recreation. Don't feel that you have to eliminate all of your fun activities to conserve your energy for work and/or family obligations. It will just increase your stress and your resentment in the long run. Many people with rheumatoid arthritis find that staying busy and concentrating on something other than arthritis boosts their sense of well-being and helps sustain their spirits during times of pain or diminished activity.

Another positive way to handle stress is to take good care of your body. A foundation of good health is like having money in a bank. You can draw upon it in times of need. Make every effort to eat a balanced diet, exercise appropriately, and get enough rest and sleep. Learn to listen to your body for physical signs of stress: If your head aches or your heart is beating fast during everyday situations, such as when you're driving or cooking dinner, you may be pushing too hard.

LEARNING TO RELAX

The ability to relax can help you relieve symptoms of stress, including tight muscles, fast and shallow breathing, fast heart rate, and high blood pressure. In addition, feeling relaxed helps you have a sense of well-being and control, which contributes to your ability to cope with stress. Learning relaxation techniques is not easy, especially if you are in pain.

If you would like to try some simple imagery and relaxation exercises, there are several listed at the end of this chapter. Again, remember that these methods take practice. Don't expect immediate results. It may be several weeks before you reap benefits from some techniques.

If You Experience Depression

Anyone who develops an illness – particularly a chronic illness such as rheumatoid arthritis – may experience psychological distress, which may manifest itself as feelings of depression and helplessness. Not everyone experiences these feelings, but if you do it is important to recognize them so you can find ways to effectively deal with these types of distress.

DEPRESSION

Everyone feels "down" or "blue" occasionally, and they may refer to these feelings as being depressed. Clinical depression, however, is a severe and prolonged feeling that can hamper your ability to function normally. If you think you may have clinical depression, you should discuss it with a doctor because there are many ways to treat this condition.

It has long been debated whether people with rheumatoid arthritis experience higher levels of depression than others without the disease. The confusion about this issue stems in part from the fact that some signs

of depression, such as fatigue and feelings of overall poor health, are also signs of rheumatoid arthritis. This confusion is related to the issue of a "rheumatoid personality," discussed earlier in this chapter, which experts do not believe to be a valid concept. Thus, many of the questionnaires designed to assess depression include "physical" rather than "psychological" problems in people who have rheumatoid arthritis, and may be interpreted to indicate that a person is depressed.

A second issue is whether depression is more common in women than in men. It is true that women tend to have higher scores on depression questionnaires, suggesting higher levels of depression. However, one possible explanation for the phenomenon is that women are more likely to recognize and acknowledge depression, as well as many other health problems, than men. It may be that actual levels of depression are similar in men and women, but there is a "reporting bias" that is picked up by the questionnaire.

Although the debate continues on these issues, it is reasonable that there might be some depression associated with the pain, fatigue, uncertainty and loss of function that people who have rheumatoid arthritis must face. There is the fear of what may or may not happen as the disease progresses – how arthritis will affect your ability to perform normal activities and to live independently. It's important to realize that depression – like arthritis – is not something to suffer through silently. It can be treated: You can talk to a qualified professional about your feelings, and you can feel better and in more control of your life.

HELPLESSNESS

Feelings of helplessness may occur when you are unable to do many of the things you used to do independently, or when you are unable to accomplish as much as you previously were able to do each day. As we mentioned at the beginning of this chapter, self-efficacy skills can be used to offset these feelings of helplessness. Results of studies have shown that people who learn to use self-efficacy skills show improvements in both their mental attitudes and their physical abilities to function. Interestingly, treatment with methotrexate and other disease-modifying drugs also is associated with an improvement in the feelings of helplessness for most people.

Personally Speaking — Stories from real people with rheumatoid arthritis

"I wonder if there is a person out there who has some golden years to their credit, has been diagnosed with rheumatoid arthritis, and who hasn't experienced this:

"I'd go into the bathroom housing the same facilities I'd been using for umpteen years, and all of a sudden they're aren't facilities anymore – they're obstacles. The appliance that set the most unique trap for me was the toilet seat, in our household referred to as the 'johnny seat.'

Vanity Works For Me
by Betty Moore, Lukeville, AZ

"Sitting down on it wasn't too much of a problem, even though at times, my knees didn't want to bend as easily as they used to, and I'd land with a thud. It was the process of getting up that was tough, beginning what I termed the 'johnny rock.' Getting up off that booby trap turned me into a contortionist, with my arthritis gnawing at my joints. My mind says, 'OK, I'm ready to get up.' Every fiber in my body told me to stand up. But there I sat. I'd get my hands braced so they could help me force myself up and off. That's where the rocking begins. I'd rock back thinking, 'This time I will push myself up and off this seat.' But somehow, it's like I have a magnet sewn onto my bottom, and the johnny seat is made of steel.

"I feel defeated, and then the ultimate motivation takes possession of me. If I can't get off this seat, I will have to call for help from my husband. All of a sudden, an extra surge of adrenaline flows through my veins, and with a very determined push with the hands and shoulders, no matter the pain, *zap!* I'm standing. Vanity – no doubt about it, it works for me."

ACTIVITY: Deep Breathing

Deep breathing is a basic technique that applies to almost all relaxation exercises. This simple technique is key to mastering the art of unwinding. Here are the steps:

1. Get as comfortable as you can. Loosen any tight clothing or jewelry, uncross your legs and arms. Close your eyes.

2. Place your hands firmly but comfortably on your stomach. This will help you feel when you are breathing properly. When you breathe correctly, your stomach expands out as you breathe in and it contracts in when you breathe out. (Many people breathe "backwards" – they tighten their stomachs when they breathe in, and relax their stomachs when they breathe out. If you're a "backwards breather," take a minute to get yourself coordinated.)

3. Inhale slowly and deeply through your nose to a count of three. Feel your stomach push against your hands? Let it expand as much as possible as you fill your lungs with air.

4. When your lungs are full, purse your lips (as if you were going to whistle) and exhale slowly through your mouth for a count of six. (Pursing your lips allows you to control how slow or fast you exhale.) Feel your stomach shrink away from your hands?

5. When your lungs feel empty, close your mouth and begin the inhale-exhale cycle again.

6. Repeat the inhale-exhale cycle three or four times at each session.

7. Whenever you're ready, slowly open your eyes and stretch.

TIP: Breathing deeply can make you feel light-headed or dizzy – especially when you are tired or hungry. It's a good idea to first practice deep breathing while you are sitting or lying down. Once you get the hang of it, deep breathing can be used anytime, anyplace.

ACTIVITY: Relaxation to Control Pain

BEGINNING PART (excerpted from "Imaginative Progressive Relaxation" technique):

First, take some time to make sure that you are in a really comfortable position. Make a quick check from head to toe to determine whether your whole body is being supported. Adjust any parts that feel uncomfortable. Try not to have legs or arms crossed, but most importantly, do what is comfortable for you.

Now, close your eyes. Become aware of your breathing. Feel the movement of your body as you breathe in and out. Breathe in slowly and exhale. On your next breath, focus on the image of breathing in good, clean air . . . and exhaling all your tensions with your breath out. Allow your breathing rhythm to pleasantly slow down. Feel as though tension is being released each time you breathe out.

MIDDLE PART:

Option 1: *"Pain Drain"* Now, feel within your body and note where you experience pain or tension. Imagine that the pain or tension is turning into a liquid substance. This heavy liquid flows down through your body and out through your fingers and toes. Allow the pain to drain from your body in a steady flow. Now, imagine that a gentle rain flows down over your head ... and further dissolves the pain ... into a liquid that continues to drain away. Enjoy the sense of comfort and well-being that follows.

Option 2: *"Disappearing Pain"* Now, notice any tension or pain that you are experiencing. Imagine that the pain takes the form of an object ... or several objects. It can be fruit, pebbles, crystals, or anything else that comes to mind. Pick each piece of pain, one at a time, and place it in a magic box.

As you drop each piece into the box, it dissolves into nothingness. Now, again survey within your body to see if any pieces remain, and you may remove them if you wish. Imagine that your body is lighter now, and allow yourself to experience a feeling of comfort and well-being. Enjoy this feeling of tranquility and repose.

Option 3: *"Healing Potion"* Now, imagine you are in a drugstore that is stocked with bottles and jars of exotic potions. Each potion has a special magical quality. Some are of pure, white light, others are lotions, balms and creams, and still others contain healing vibrations. As you survey the many potions, choose one that appeals to you. It may even have your name on the container. Open the container and cover your body with that magical potion. As you apply it, let any pain or tension slowly melt away, leaving you with a feeling of comfort and well-being. Imagine that you place the container in a special spot and that it continually renews its contents for future use.

Option 4: *"Leaving Pain Behind"* Imagine that you are dreaming now. Although your body stays in the same position, imagine that you are gently leaving it. ... As you leave your body, notice that you have also left your tension and pain behind. Pick a special spot to visit, one that brings pleasure and a feeling of well-being. Notice how your dreamlike body feels as you visit this special place. Linger here for a while ... and when you feel ready, return to your position in alignment with your body. When you open your eyes, retain the freedom from tension and pain, and continue to experience a sense of comfort and well-being.

END PART:

Whenever you are ready, slowly stretch and open your eyes.

Adapted from *The ROM Dance,* a range-of-motion and relaxation program, Diane Harlowe and Patricia Yu, 1992. Published by St. Mary's Hospital Medical Center, Madison, WI. Materials available from The ROM Dance, P.O. Box 3332, Madison, WI 53709. 800/488-4940.

ACTIVITY: Guided-Imagery Smorgasbord

Think of guided imagery as a daydream with a tour guide. By diverting your attention away from stress, guided imagery takes your mind on a mini-vacation. Use your imagination to transport yourself to a more peaceful place. It's up to you to choose where. For some people the most relaxing place is the seashore; for others it's the mountains. Pick your mind's ideal vacation spot, and go there. The following exercise teaches you how to focus on relaxing in your choice of desirable, stress-free locations. Again, have a friend read the exercise to you – or record it yourself and play it back as you imagine.

BEGINNING RITUAL:

Get as comfortable as you can, feet slightly apart, arms resting at your sides. Now close your eyes. Take a slow deep breath in through your nose and slowly exhale through your mouth. Again, take a deep breath in . . . and slowly exhale. Continue to breath slowly and deeply. Notice yourself getting more and more relaxed. Let all your tension melt away.

MIDDLE PART:

Option 1: *"Sea"* Your body is very heavy, at ease and warm. . . Listen to your heart . . . it is beating steadily . . . and regularly. . . As you listen to your heart . . . you feel its beat . . . in your whole body . . . It feels as though you are on a boat . . . on a quiet calm sea . . . with the water lapping against the sides . . .

You're inhaling and exhaling like the waves. . . . They are gently rocking you. . . The rocking continues in your mind . . . and as you rock . . . one after the other the negative emotions are dropping out of you . . . frustration . . . sorrow . . . depression . . . heartache . . . worries . . . resentment. . . You feel serene and content . . .

You feel so wonderful you'd like the whole world to enjoy it with you . . . and out of the depths of your heart rises a great lightness . . . and you feel it flow in a continuous steady stream through your whole body . . . and all the time you feel lighter . . . and lighter . . .

Adapted from the *Arthritis Movement Workshop Leader's Manual*, Arthritis Foundation, Arizona Chapter.

Option 2: *"Pine Forest"* Imagine in as much detail as possible that you are sitting comfortably in a chair or hammock in the middle of a beautiful pine forest. . . Enjoy the fresh, cool, clean, fragrant air. . . What a pleasure it is to breathe! . . . Imagine the gentle, cool breeze as it touches your skin.

You are sitting comfortably, feeling peaceful and calm. . . As you casually look around, you are impressed by the beauty of the tall pine trees with their rich brown bark . . . and graceful feathery green branches. You notice the pinecones on the branches. . . . You watch the leaves of the aspen trees dancing in the wind. The ground interests you with its rich brown dirt covered with pine needles and leaves . . . and its robust, earthy aroma.

You hear birds calling . . . and a woodpecker at work in the distance. . . You notice a small clearing in the forest. The clearing is covered with green grass and beautiful wildflowers of all types and colors. You see butterflies around the flowers. You are at peace in your pine forest, sitting comfortably, feeling relaxed and calm . . . appreciating the wonders of nature . . . and of being alive.

Adapted from the *Multiple Sclerosis Self-Help Course Leader's Guide* by Katalina McGlone, 1984.

Option 3: *"Ocean Beach"* Imagine that you are at the ocean. . . . You are sitting comfortably on the beach under the shade of a large beach umbrella. . . . Feel the warm sand under you . . . and the warm, comfortable air around you . . . and the refreshing, soft breeze blowing through your hair. . . Feel the warm moisture in the air upon your face. . . Notice the smell of the ocean . . . Imagine how beautiful, brilliantly blue the sky is . . .

You're sitting on the beach ... feeling calm ... peaceful ... relaxed ... comfortable.... You are watching the waves ... as they grow and break ... mesmerized as they go in and out from the shore... You can hear the thundering of the waves as they break... The only other sounds are those of the seagulls...

Notice how peaceful you feel ... sitting on the beach ... feeling in harmony with nature.

Adapted from the *Systemic Lupus Erythematosus Self-Help Course Leader's Manual* – Katalina McGlone, 1984.

Option 4: *"Floating in Space"* Imagine you are standing on a mat in front of an elevator. The doors open, you step in and watch the numbers slowly change: 1, 2, 3, 4, 5, 6, 7, 8, 9, 10. The doors open, and you step out into deep, dark outer space. Feel yourself floating weightlessly, drifting, being very light. See the pure, velvety deep blue color of space all around you. Look at the earth, small and green-blue ... Imagine stars and planets moving past you in the distance. Imagine yourself moving towards a space of diffuse white light, as bright and ethereal as a distant star ... As you approach this light, it increases in size until you feel yourself surrounded by its glow. Being in the light, you feel that you are bathed in feelings of tranquility and well-being.

If disturbing thoughts or feelings enter your mind as you are in this place, allow them to pass by you, just as you imagine planets and stars passing by you on this voyage. Let these thoughts and feelings fade into the distance, leaving them behind you in the same way that you might imagine a comet disappearing over the horizon.

Enjoy the peaceful feelings of this place... Slowly float out of the white light, imagining that it has filled your body and you are carrying it with you. Then float back past the stars and planets through the deep velvety blue-black space to the elevator. Step back in, see the doors close, watch the numbers change: 10, 9, 8, 7, 6, 5, 4, 3, 2, 1. The doors open and you are back on your mat. Feel your body on the mat.

Adapted from the *Arthritis Movement Workshop Leader's Manual*, Arthritis Foundation, Arizona Chapter.

Option 5: *"Memory and Fantasy"* In this relaxation exercise, remember a past experience – or create a new one – with your imagination. Imagine yourself in an environment where you feel secure, comfortable and relaxed. This can be a place you remember ... a fantasy you are creating ... or a mixture of memory and imagination. Simply experience whatever comes to you. Sometimes the environment will change during the exercise, and sometimes it will remain the same.

Place yourself in this environment and note how you are positioned ... standing ... sitting ... or lying down. In this secure, comfortable, relaxed environment, look around you. Take in the panorama of colors, forms and textures. If you are outside or can see outside ... note the season ... time of day or night ... and the weather. Look all around you ... in front ... behind ... both sides ... above ... and below you. Look at the sky or ceiling ... the ground or floor ... in the distance ... and up close. Are there other people here? Take in all you wish to see. What sounds come to you? Listen for sounds in the distance ... up close ... all around you. From what directions do the sounds come?

In this secure, relaxed and comfortable environment ... is there anything that you can smell? If something to drink or eat presents itself ... taste it fully and note its texture in your mouth. Is there anything or anybody you are touching? How does it feel?

How does the environment around you feel physically? ...Warm or cool? ...Damp or dry? Do you feel movement in the air? How does it feel emotionally? ...How do you feel inside in this environment?

Once again, take in the sights around you... They may have changed. Note the sounds ... smells ... tastes ... and sights. Focus on emotional feelings ... the feelings inside.

Adapted from *The ROM Dance*, a range-of-motion and relaxation program, Diane Harlowe and Patricia Yu, 1992. Materials available from The ROM Dance, P.O. Box 3332, Madison, WI 53709. 800/488-4940.

Option 6: *"Water Fantasy"* Imagine that you are immersed in water, perhaps in your bathtub... in a lake ... swimming pool ... or even a whirlpool bath. Imagine that the water is the perfect temperature ... just warm enough so that every muscle in your body feels as supple and flowing as the very water itself. Experience the water flowing around and coming into contact with each part of you. As it does this, it melts away deeper levels of tension ... leaving your whole body feeling cleansed and drained of all tension.

Let yourself stay in this wonderful water for a while, letting go of deeper and deeper levels of tension ... and allowing yourself to feel more and more relaxed.

Adapted from *The ROM Dance*.

END PART:

(Silence) ...You may go back to this place whenever you want, simply by sitting quietly and remembering this place in as much detail as possible....Whenever you are ready, move your fingers, wiggle your toes, and come back to this world feeling refreshed and invigorated.

Build up your resistance to stress. Stress can have a negative effect on your body. Taking good care of your body can help you build up resistance to stress. Ways to take good care of your body include:

- eating a balanced diet
- exercising
- avoiding drugs and alcohol
- getting enough rest and sleep
- saving energy by pacing your activities
- accentuating the positive.

Incorporate the relaxation techniques you've learned in this chapter into your daily life and you'll reap rewards. Managing your stress — whether or not you have rheumatoid arthritis — can lessen pain and increase good living.

Chapter 14

Physical Challenges:

Managing the Ups and Downs

Having rheumatoid arthritis can create many physical challenges in your daily life. Although treatments for arthritis have improved dramatically in the last 15 years, dealing with daily morning stiffness or occasional flares can seem daunting. Also, you may wonder what you can do to save wear and tear on your joints.

In this chapter, we will discuss some tips and techniques to help you deal with the physical side of rheumatoid arthritis: acute and chronic pain, as well as the physical limitations that can result from stiffness and joint damage.

Your overall program for managing rheumatoid arthritis contributes to lessening pain, so it's important to commit to regular exercise, balancing activity with rest and respecting your limits. Understanding your limits does not mean that you give in to your pain; rather, you are finding ways to manage it.

Pain for people with rheumatoid arthritis may have several causes that should be recognized, because solving the problem may involve different approaches.

• **Inflammation.** This process causes your joints to swell and become red.

• **Damage to joint tissues.** Damage may be due to the disease process of rheumatoid arthritis, or from stress or pressure on the joints.

• **Muscle tightness or fibromyalgia.** Inflammation of the joints may lead to muscle weakness or stiffness at times. Some people with rheumatoid arthritis also experience fibromyalgia (see Chapter 5), marked by widespread muscle pain.

Pain is generally amplified by fatigue and poor sleep, both common in people with rheumatoid arthritis. Feelings of depression or helplessness can lower your pain threshold, making you more vulnerable to pain.

While you are no stranger to pain, it doesn't have to dominate your life. Most people experience good days and bad days. Pain management specialists emphasize that a healthy approach to coping with pain can help you maximize your good days and minimize the pain you feel on bad days. Whether dealing with acute pain during a flare or ongoing, everyday pain, you can learn to help yourself by thinking about your relationship to pain and applying some of the techniques in this chapter that appeal to you.

One woman with rheumatoid arthritis said she had learned to remind herself during pain episodes that her body was sick, but her mind was not. By using your mind – to implement relaxation techniques or to organize daily chores more efficiently – you can become your own best ally in managing pain.

What Is Pain?

When your body is injured in any way, the nerves of your damaged tissue trigger the release of chemicals. These chemicals relay messages to your brain, causing the unpleasant sensations we call pain. There are many causes of pain, as diverse as trauma and inflammation. Pain may be sharp or dull, chronic or acute, localized (felt in only one or two places) or generalized (felt through-

---

Non-Drug Strategies for Closing the Gate on Pain

- Heat or cold treatments. Usually applied directly to the site of pain; heat may be more useful for chronic pain, whereas cold packs provide relief from acute pain.

- Positive attitude and thoughts. Consciously switching to positive thoughts can distract your brain from feeling pain (see Chapter 13).

- Exercise. Keeping your joints and muscles moving helps improve your general fitness level and can decrease pain.

- Relaxation techniques. You can train your muscles to relax and your thoughts to slow down by using these techniques, which include deep breathing, guided imagery and visualization, among others.

- Massage. When done properly, this method can relax your muscles and help you let go of tension.

- Electrical stimulation. Delivered through a small device called transcutaneous electrical nerve stimulation (TENS), it blocks pain by stimulating large nerve fibers, or by causing the release of endorphins. TENS is usually prescribed by your doctor or physical therapist.

- Topical lotions. These are applied directly to the skin over the painful muscle or joint. They may contain salicylates or capsaicin, which decrease sensitivity to pain.

- Acupuncture. Considered a complementary or nontraditional therapy, acupuncture is the practice of inserting fine needles into the body along special points called "meridians" to relieve pain (see Chapter 17 on complementary and alternative therapies).

- Sense of humor. Many studies have demonstrated that humor can help bolster the immune system and increase the ability to handle pain.

out the body). In rheumatoid arthritis, pain may be caused by *synovitis*, or inflammation of the synovial membrane surrounding the joint. The result is swelling and tenderness.

Individual responses to pain vary widely. What one person can barely feel, another can hardly tolerate. This is one reason your doctor must rely on your reports of pain when examining you and when prescribing pain medications. Pain can be measured on various types of scales, such as a *visual analogue scale*, which asks you to rate your pain on a scale of 0 to 10 (or 0 to 100), with zero indicating "no pain" and 10 (or 100) being "pain as bad as it can be." Keeping track of your pain scores over time can help you and your doctor see how your disease is progressing and whether your pain medications and coping strategies are working.

THE "GATE" THEORY OF PAIN

Your nervous system plays an important role in how you experience pain. You may have heard reports about people with traumatic injuries feeling no pain immediately after an accident occurred. Somehow the nervous system blocks the pain signals by producing chemicals called *endorphins* to lead to a good feeling. Other situations can trigger production of endorphins, such as the so-called "runner's high," which describes the euphoria experienced by runners during their physical exertion.

So why is it that some pain signals get blocked? According to one theory, known as the *gate control theory of pain*, when pain sig-

nals reach the nervous system, they stimulate a group of nerve cells that form a "pain pool." Upon reaching a certain level of activity, a virtual gate opens up, allowing the pain signals to proceed to higher centers in the brain. However, the gate can also be closed by certain signals. For example, medications such as morphine and other narcotics act as synthetic endorphins that block the pain signal, so the gate does not open.

Research has shown that, in addition to pain medication, there are nondrug factors that can be used to close the pain gate. Some or all of the strategies listed in the box on page 132 may be useful to you in dealing with the pain of rheumatoid arthritis. Many of them are discussed at greater length in this chapter or the chapters that follow.

Knowing what closes the pain gate can help you feel more in control and create your own plan of action to deal with pain. You should be aware that, just as certain factors can close the pain gate, others can open it, making you feel more pain. Some of these factors, such as a sudden increase in inflammatory activity (a flare) are beyond your control. But there are other factors that you *can* control, at least in part. These include:

- **Prolonged stress or anxiety.**
- **Obsessing about pain and negative thoughts.**
- **Too little physical activity.**
- **Too much physical activity or exertion.**
- **Overindulgence in alcohol.**
- **Overuse of pain medications.**

"GRIN AND BEAR IT" DOES NOT WORK

There may be times when you think that the best strategy for dealing with pain is to simply ignore it. Although this approach may work for short periods – say, as you override pain in your hands to finish typing a document – it is rarely wise to ignore or deny pain for long periods of time. Remember that pain is a signal that something is not right inside your body.

Research suggests that chemicals released by your body when you are feeling pain can actually make the inflammation of rheumatoid arthritis worse. The only good thing about pain is that it signals you that something is wrong. There is no advantage to feeling pain over long periods. Don't be afraid to take medications to relieve your pain.

Just because others cannot see your pain does not mean you are not justified in addressing it. If you have concerns about becoming dependent on pain medication, speak to your doctor. Most of the drugs prescribed for pain relief are not addictive, and even potentially addictive drugs usually do not lead to chemical dependence in people who experience severe pain.

Managing a Flare

Although rheumatoid arthritis is a chronic disease, you can have acute episodes of pain and inflammation, known as *flares*. Flares may be seen after infections, or after highly stressful situations. Often, however, it is not clear what triggers a flare. You may have long periods of time when your rheumatoid arthritis is quiet, or in remission. Then, suddenly, the inflammation becomes more active and you have an arthritis flare.

Flares can be alarming, not only because of the pain, but because of their unpredictability. You may feel discouraged or afraid of further damage to your joints. You sometimes wonder whether something you did may have caused the flare.

What can you do to combat these feelings? Remember that you have a range of tools in your arsenal to address pain – from asking your doctor to increase your pain medications, to applying cold packs or practicing deep breathing techniques. Also, remember that flares do calm down. You may want to think about how you will handle the inevitable "bad days" and flares before you experience them. Just as regular fire drills help people deal with real emergencies, preparing for a flare can help you jump into action when it happens.

Discuss a plan of action with your doctor. One possible approach would be to adjust your medications temporarily while the disease is unusually active. This will not only relieve some of the pain associated with a flare; it will also help minimize any damage that may occur from unchecked inflammation.

Be aware that your medications may not control the flare right away, even if your dosages are increased. Or they may only have a limited effect on your flare. Of course you and your doctors should be in agreement about possible increases in your medications, or even additions of new medications at the time of a flare. Many doctors will review such a plan for a flare that can be implemented when needed without permission from the doctor.

The following is a list of some other steps that you may want to incorporate in your plan of action. Remember, some techniques work better for some people than others. Try a few of these, and if they don't work for you, discard them and try others.

- **Balance periods of activity with periods of rest.** Although more rest can help during a flare, you probably do not need to abandon your regular activities, work or exercise program. A doctor or physical therapist can help you modify your program when you experience a flare. Spending long periods of time in bed is counterproductive – it usually will prolong your pain. Instead, try to intersperse periods of rest with some light activity. Finally, to keep joints from becoming stiff, move them through the full range of motion possible, gradually increasing your range as the flare subsides.

Personally Speaking   Stories from real people with rheumatoid arthritis

"In 1994, I noticed a strange soreness and stiffness in my hands, then in my wrists and ankles. In less than a year, every joint was engulfed in pain. I found it difficult to continue the simple tasks of living – caring for myself and my family, sleeping, working. They all became almost impossible for me. It hurt just to move. I was living, but I did not feel *alive*. To control the pain, I was on many medications, some with dangerous side effects.

The Christmas Gift in a Prescription Bottle
by Stacy White-Werner,
Perry, MI

"Despite medications and therapies, I continued to get worse. Then, in December 1998, I started taking the drug *Enbrel*. I call it my Christmas gift. I have been on this medication since then, and the results are fantastic. I am not in remission, but I am close. I feel stronger every day. I am slowly getting my life back. I am continuing the education that I had put off. I feel like a wife and mother again. When I can completely control my symptoms, I plan on returning to work.

"In addition to medications, I also try to stay active and eat a well-balanced diet. My friends and family are also part of my healing process. Without their love and support, it would be tough to face life with rheumatoid arthritis. They give me the added strength to keep living in spite of it. The other way I cope is by keeping a positive outlook. This is my life, and my body. I'm not going to let rheumatoid arthritis steal any more of it away from me."

- **Have a plan to deal with your obligations.** Have a contingency plan both for work obligations and family obligations. At work, try to arrange for coverage, work fewer hours per week or bring work home. Discuss your plan with supervisors and co-workers ahead of time, and assure them of your commitment. At home, plan to apportion a few extra jobs among family members, and make sure everyone knows what they are expected to do to keep things running smoothly.

- **Communicate with your family and friends.** The time to let your family and friends know that you may need more help is when things are going well. When a flare occurs, if someone volunteers to help you, give them a specific job. Otherwise, well-intentioned offers of assistance go unused. There may be other sources of help available to you as well, such as members of your religious institution or community volunteer organizations.

- **Apply a hot or cold pack to inflamed joints.** Some people find hot or cold packs helpful – different people may prefer one or the other. Although heat can theoretically make inflammation worse, because it tends to increase blood flow and nerve sensitivity, some people find a warm pack soothing and pain relieving. Others get great benefit from cold, which decreases blood flow to the inflamed area and decreases inflammation and muscle spasm. It can provide temporary relief from acute pain. You can buy warm and cold packs from a drugstore or medical supply outlet, or you can use a hot water bottle or simply wrap a towel around a bag of frozen vegetables (to avoid ice burn, never place the ice pack directly on your skin). The pack should be comfortable to the contours of the joint. Leave the pack on the area for about 10 minutes, then remove it for an equal amount of time. Some people even prefer warm packs for certain joints and cold packs for other joints. You will learn your own preferences through trial and error.

- **Practice relaxation or mind-diversion techniques.** These techniques work best when you practice them on a regular basis. Even though relaxation may not directly reduce your pain, it can minimize stress, which is a factor shown to amplify pain.

Many other techniques are available. When you find those that work for you, write them down and use them as often as needed – particularly when you experience a bad day or a flare of your rheumatoid arthritis.

Managing Chronic Pain

Chronic pain – defined as pain that lasts longer than a few months – can be even more challenging to deal with than acute pain. You probably know from experience that a flare does not last, and you will feel better. However, handling the chronic pain and stiffness that go on day after day can lead to fatigue, discouragement and even depression. For some people with rheumatoid arthritis, pain becomes a constant companion. It's important to learn to manage your chronic pain, so that you do not become its victim.

Some of the techniques that work for acute flares, such as relaxation, meditation and guided imagery, are also helpful in reducing or minimizing chronic pain. One goal of these approaches is to train your brain and body to focus on positive images, thus directing your attention away from your pain. The benefits seem to build over time, so practice them on a regular basis.

In addition, treatments involving heat or cold can provide soothing relief for stiff joints and tired muscles. There are many forms of these therapies. Experiment with the warming ideas in the box below to find out which ones work best for you.

Warming Techniques

- Take a long and very warm shower first thing in the morning to ease morning stiffness.
- Soak in a warm bath or whirlpool.
- Buy a moist heat pad from the drugstore, or make one at home by putting a wet wash cloth in a freezer bag and heating it in the microwave for one minute. Wrap the hot pack in a towel and place it over the affected area for 15 to 20 minutes.
- To soothe stiff and painful joints in your hands, apply mineral oil to your hands, put on rubber dishwashing gloves, and place your hands in hot tap water for 5 to 10 minutes.
- Incorporate other warming elements into your daily routines, such as warming your clothes in the dryer before dressing or using an electric blanket and turning it up before getting out of bed.

A physical therapist can give you many additional ideas for using heat to temporarily relieve pain and ease stiffness.

Avoiding Joint Pain and Damage

Managing pain should be proactive, instead of simply being reactive. In other words, you should try to manage pain at its beginning and not wait for it to become severe. Likewise, you can reduce the day-to-day stresses placed on joints in everyday activities to avoid damage.

In addition to regular exercise, you can learn many ways to use your body to reduce joint stress. You can avoid trying to open tight-fitting jars and performing twisting motions on the dance floor. Learning to listen to your body's signals when you need to rest can also reduce pain, because energy reserves can enhance your abilities to cope with pain. Some of the most common techniques are described here, along with examples.

BODY MECHANICS OR ERGONOMICS

Body mechanics is the use of proper techniques for bending, lifting, reaching, sitting and standing. The idea is always to use the largest and most stable joints to do the work. This spreads out the load and lessens stress on weaker joints, or those with more disease involvement.

- **Use your palms.** When you lift or carry things, use the palms of both hands instead of your fingers.
- **Use large muscles.** If you carry a purse, put it over your shoulder or consider switching to a back pack or fanny pack.

- **Lift with your legs.** When lifting something low or on the ground, always bend your knees and lift by straightening your legs.
- **Stand up properly.** To get up from a chair, slide forward to the chair's edge and place your feet flat on the floor. Lean forward, then push down with your palms (not your fingers) on the arms or seat of the chair. Stand up by straightening your hips and knees.
- **Practice good posture.** When standing, practice good posture by imagining a straight line that connects your ears, shoulders, hips, knees and heels. Knees should be slightly bent, stomach and buttocks tucked in, and shoulders back.
- **Use props.** Put some pillows on a chair, and consider using a raised toilet seat, to help you get up and down more easily.

BALANCING REST AND ACTIVITY

Both work and leisure activities are important. The trick is in balancing them. Moderation should be your motto, especially when your arthritis is more active.

- **Pace yourself.** Take short breaks and alternate heavy and light activities during the day.
- **Don't set unrealistic goals.** Make a "to do" list that isn't too long – and don't add to it.
- **Keep active.** Too much rest is not good for your joints either. Even on days when you are tired or stiff, try to do some exercise. By increasing your level of fitness, you will actually have more energy and less pain.

- **Know when to take breaks.** Don't wait for the physical signals of pain before you rest.

ORGANIZE AND SIMPLIFY YOUR LIFE

We would all like to be more organized and able to streamline our daily routines. It's an especially good idea if you have rheumatoid arthritis, because the energy you save at work by having everything handy at your desk may mean the difference between coming home exhausted and being able to enjoy the evening. You may expect some guidance from health professionals to help you organize your life, but you can get started by using a few simple ideas.

- **Keep tools handy.** If you work, keep all equipment and tools within easy reach and at a comfortable level. Use a lazy Susan or storage bins to keep supplies handy.
- **Simplify cleaning.** Streamline cleaning chores by using some of the new "all in one" cleaning products, or those that require little or no scrubbing. Don't try to clean everything in one day – rotate the tasks over the course of the week instead.
- **Plan ahead.** When cooking, put all necessary tools and ingredients on the counter before you start to minimize trips to the pantry and refrigerator. Use convenience foods – such as chicken that is precooked and cubed – to save energy and wear and tear on joints.
- **Organize your errands.** If your bank is near the dry cleaner, make one trip instead of two.

Where to Purchase Self-Help Devices

The companies listed below are manufacturers of ergonomic office equipment and daily living equipment. You may request catalogs, and may purchase directly from the company or through your physical therapist, occupational therapist or health-care provider.

This list is by no means complete, but it may give you a good place to begin searching for useful products. Consult a physical or occupational therapist or speak to your doctor to find more sources of self-help or assistive devices.

There is also a non-profit organization called Illinois Assistive Technology Project, that helps people find assistive devices and maintains lists of companies that sell them. This Illinois organization can provide information specific to your state: **Illinois Assistive Technology Project** • 1 West Old State Capitol Plaza • Suite 100 • Springfield, IL 62701 • 800/852-5110 (in Illinois Only) • 217/522-7985 • www.iltech.org

---

ERGONOMIC OFFICE EQUIPMENT
Ergonomic Solutions
129 N. Sylvan Drive • Mundelein, IL 60060-4949
(800) 755-4950 • www.goergo.com
Call to obtain a catalog of products, including the Ergo rest and other arm supports, to make computer keyboarding easier.

Ergo Source
P.O. Box 695 • Wayzata, MN 55391
(800) 969-4374
Leave a message requesting company literature. Products include office accessories, forearm supports, foot rests and adjustable work surfaces.

DAILY LIVING EQUIPMENT
Smith and Nephew
P.O. Box 1005 • Germantown, WI 53022
(800) 558-8633 • www.smith-nephew.com
Upon request, this company will send you its "Activities for Daily Living" catalog.

North Coast Medical
Consumer Products Division
18305 Sutter Blvd. • Morgan Hill, CA 95037
(800) 235-7054
NCM offers a "Return to Fitness" catalog, featuring products for physical therapy and rehabilitation.

Aids for Arthritis, Inc.
35 Wakefield Drive • Medford, NJ 08055
(800) 654-0707
Leave a message with your name and address, and the company will send you its "Self-Help Products" catalog.

Mature Smart
1788 West Cherry St. • Jesup, GA 31545
800/720-6278 • www.maturesmart.com
Request a copy of this company's daily living products catalog, which includes a section on "Arthritis Aids."

Sears Home HealthCare
3737 Grader Street, Suite 110 • Garland, TX 75041
(800) 326-1750
Upon request, Sears will send you a copy of its home health-care products catalog.

Kinsman Enterprises
P.O. Box 364 • Benton, IL 62812
(618) 439-0519
This company deals with hospitals, providers and consumers, and charges the same price to all. Call for an activities of daily-living products catalog.

SELF-HELP DEVICES

When you're tired, stiff or in a hurry, self-help devices can make tasks easier on your joints and more efficient for you. These products, which range from the simple to the elaborate, help keep joints in the best position for function, provide leverage when needed, and extend your range of motion. The companies listed in the box on page 139 are some of the many who sell self-help devices. Simple devices, such as jar openers, reachers and easy-grip utensils can be purchased at many hardware or medical supply stores.

- **In the bedroom.** When dressing, zipper pulls and buttoning aids can help you fasten clothing. Or you can choose to wear clothing with *Velcro* fasteners when available. A long-handled shoehorn lets you extend your reach without bending.
- **In the kitchen.** In the kitchen, appliances such as electric can openers and food processors make work easier. Reachers (long-handled tools with a gripping mechanism) can be used to retrieve items stored high or low. Built-up handles and grips make utensils easier to grasp and put less stress on finger joints. Install a fixed jar opener, or keep a rubber jar opener in the kitchen.

- **In the bathroom.** Tub bars and handrails provide additional stability and security when getting into and out of the bath or shower. These are a must if you have problems with balance. Faucet levers or tap turners are available if your grip is weak. A raised toilet seat can make it easier to sit down and get up from the toilet.
- **In the office.** In the work environment, many devices and modifications are available, from adjustable-height chairs and work surfaces to telephones with large push buttons and a special built-up headset. If you are facing work modifications, you will probably want to see an occupational therapist. He or she can help you make changes and obtain the devices you need.
- **At play.** Leisure activities can still be enjoyable through the use of assistive devices such as kneelers and light-weight hoses for gardening, "no-hands" frames for quilting or embroidery, and card holders and shufflers for card games, to name just a few.
- **In the car.** When driving, a wide key holder can make it much easier to turn on the ignition. A gas cap opener can help when filling the tank at the gas station.

Chapter 15

Exercise:

The Importance of Getting Physical

If you have rheumatoid arthritis, you may be confused about exercise. Perhaps someone has told you that you should rest or protect your joints – and they're right. You do need to take extra care of joints that are actively inflamed. However, that does not mean you should avoid exercise. As you will see, exercise can be an important part of your self-management plan. Believe it or not, it can also be an important way to protect your joints.

In this chapter, we will discuss some of the ways that regular exercise can benefit people with rheumatoid arthritis. We will also review the types of exercises that should be part of your routine, and will even include some simple exercises to get you started.

Why exercise? Some kind of exercise is good for almost everyone, but research has shown that it can be especially helpful for people with rheumatoid arthritis. The disease process – and the damage it causes – may lead to limited joint range of motion, decreased muscle strength and endurance, and general deconditioning. Appropriate and regular exercise can lead to improvement in these areas; it also reduces pain, fatigue and depression. Some researchers have even shown that regular aerobic exercise can reduce joint swelling in people with rheumatoid arthritis.

What if I Don't Exercise?

When you're tired and your body hurts, you may not feel like exercising. It's all too easy to put off exercising because it "uses up energy" you need to complete your other daily activities. However, as the old saying goes, "If you don't use it, you lose it." Unused joints, bones and muscles deteriorate quickly. Long periods of inactivity can lead to weakness, stiffness, increased fatigue, poor appetite, constipation, increased blood pressure, obesity, osteoporosis, and heightened sensitivity to pain, anxiety and depression. Collectively, these results of inactivity are

Benefits of Regular Exercise

Keeps your body from becoming too stiff

Keeps your muscles strong

Keeps bone and cartilage tissue strong and healthy

Improves ability to do daily activities

Gives you more energy

Helps you sleep better

Helps control weight gain

Makes your heart stronger and improves cardiovascular health

Provides an outlet for stress and tension

Decreases depression and anxiety

Releases endorphins (your body's natural pain relievers)

Improves self-esteem and provides a sense of well-being

known as *deconditioning*. And, as the diagram on page 143 shows, deconditioning then leads to further pain, in a continuing cycle.

How does the cycle work? If you do not exercise, your muscles become smaller and weaker, and they are less able to support and protect you. You have less stamina and daily activities become more difficult. This loss of function and independence can increase your level of stress, which in turn creates muscle tension, leading to more pain, and so on through the cycle. Exercise is one of the prime weapons used to break this cycle.

Luckily, it has been shown that regular exercise actually *increases* the amount of energy you have. Participating in a regular exercise program is a great way to feel better and move more comfortably with less pain.

Making a Commitment To Exercise

The idea of starting an exercise program can be intimidating, particularly if you've never been very active. Just keep in mind that you should start slowly. Do whatever you can at first. As you become stronger and your endurance increases, you will be able to exercise longer and more strenuously.

One of the toughest parts of exercise is just getting started. But the effort you put into starting and maintaining a regular exercise program will come back to you many times over in terms of better health, less pain and improved mental outlook. Once you begin to enjoy the benefits of exercise, your body will become more conditioned, and you will begin to look forward to your workouts.

The following list provides some ideas to help you get started and stay motivated. Use the ideas that make sense for your personality and situation.

• **Get a physical assessment.** See a doctor or physical therapist for an assessment of your exercise and joint protection needs.

This will help you understand the reasons for exercise and set reasonable goals.

• **Set realistic exercise goals.** You may even sign a contract with yourself. Write down what you plan to do and when you plan to do it. You could have someone else "witness" the contract to help keep you motivated.

• **Make exercise a routine.** You may try to exercise at the same time each day so that it becomes a part of your routine. Try linking the time to something else: for example, after your morning shower, before lunch or after reading the newspaper.

• **Stay in the habit.** Do some exercise every day. Extra physical activity can add to improving your physical conditioning. When you feel up to it, incorporate a little extra movement into your normal routines, such as walking up the stairs instead of using an elevator.

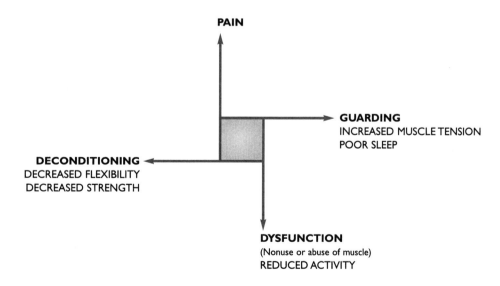

A VICIOUS CYCLE: PAIN, GUARDING, DYSFUNCTION AND DECONDITIONING

• **Make an effort every day.** On days that you have pain or you don't feel motivated, it is important to make some effort – even if you just do some gentle stretching or range-of-motion exercises.

• **Add variety.** Vary the type of exercises you do to keep from getting bored. Try doing some exercises, such as range-of-motion or muscle conditioning exercises, to music. Try rotating other exercises. For example, you could walk three days a week, swim twice and attend an arthritis exercise class twice. Ask a friend or family member to join you in a regular exercise routine. You can help motivate each other, and make exercise something social. If you make it fun, you'll be much more likely to stick with it.

• **Keep track of your progress and enjoy your successes.** There are many ways to monitor the effectiveness of your fitness program. Your doctor or health professional may notice decreased stiffness or improved gait. You will probably be able to see other benefits, such as less fatigue, less pain and decreased stress, for yourself.

Fitness Exercises: A Quick Reference Guide

Type	Suggested Uses	Benefits
Flexibility	Daily routine Get in shape for strengthening/aerobics Aerobics warm-up As needed for comfort	Flexibility Comfort Joint health Ease daily activity Relaxation
Strength	Every-other-day routine With flexibility exercise With flexibility and aerobic for total fitness program Combine upper/lower-body exercises	Protect joints Ease daily activity Relieve pain Reduce fatigue Increase endurance
Aerobic	Every-other-day routine Short sessions several times daily Alternate brisk exercise with slow exercise to build up total duration of aerobic activity	General health Increase energy Weight control Improve mood Increase stamina Lower blood pressure Strengthen bone Relaxation

Choosing the Right Moves

We hope we've convinced you that exercise is important, and important for you. But you may wonder what kinds of exercise you should include in your daily routine. Different people enjoy different types of exercises – and different people with rheumatoid arthritis have different levels of joint involvement, disease course or level of inflammatory activity.

When you are starting out, your first contact may be with a health professional – a doctor, physical therapist, trainer or exercise therapist. He or she may have a list of recommended exercises, and may give you explanatory diagrams. A complete exercise program to improve physical fitness may include exercises for flexibility, muscle strength, endurance and cardiovascular fitness. How you combine these types of exercise depends on your current capacities, exercise experience, the goals you want to accomplish, and most of all, what you like to do. To become a successful exercise self-manager, you need to discover which types of exercise are best for you and use them to meet your goals.

FLEXIBILITY (STRETCHING) EXERCISES

Flexibility exercises are intended to help keep your muscles stretched out and your joints moving freely. They can be thought of as a foundation of your exercise program, because flexibility is necessary for comfortable movement during exercise and daily activities. It also helps reduce the risk of sprains and strains.

Flexibility exercises are also referred to as range-of-motion and stretching exercises. They should be done gently and smoothly, usually every day. You may be familiar with this type of exercise as a "warm up," because it is usually recommended before performing any more vigorous type of exercise.

If you have been inactive for a while, or if you have stopped exercising temporarily because of your arthritis, these exercises are a good way to begin your fitness program. You can start by building a routine of 15 minutes of flexibility exercises. When you are able to do 15 continuous minutes, you should have the motion and endurance needed to begin adding strengthening and aerobic exercise to your program. Some sample flexibility exercises are included at the end of this chapter.

For people with rheumatoid arthritis, stiffness in the morning can be a big problem. Doing gentle flexibility exercises before getting up or during a hot bath or shower may help joints "loosen up." However, doing them later in the day may be more comfortable for many people with rheumatoid arthritis and may reduce fatigue.

STRENGTHENING EXERCISES

Exercises that increase muscle strength and endurance are the second important component of your fitness program. Joint swelling and pain can weaken muscles, as can disuse due to stiffness and pain. If you have arthritis, strong muscles are needed to climb stairs, walk safely, lift and reach. Strong muscles are important to help absorb shock, support joints and protect you from injury.

Strengthening exercises (also called resistance exercises) make your muscles work harder by adding weight or resistance to movement. There are two types: isometric and isotonic. In *isometric* exercises, you tighten your muscles without moving your joints. This helps build the muscles around your joints. In *isotonic* exercises, you move your joints to strengthen your muscles. For example, straightening your knee while sitting in a chair is an isotonic exercise that helps strengthen your thigh muscle. Flexibility

Recommended Heart Rate Ranges

Age	Heart Rate Range (60% - 75% of Age-Predicted Maximum Heart Rate)	10-Second Count
20	120 – 150	20 – 25
25	117 – 146	19 – 24
30	114 – 143	19 – 24
35	111 – 139	18 – 23
40	108 – 135	18 – 23
45	105 – 131	17 – 22
50	102 – 128	17 – 21
55	99 – 124	16 – 21
60	96 – 120	16 – 20
65	93 – 116	15 – 19
70	90 – 113	15 – 19
75	87 – 109	14 – 18
80	84 – 105	14 – 18
85	81 – 101	13 – 17
90	78 – 98	13 – 16

exercises can become strengthening exercises when you increase the speed, increase the number of repetitions, or add weight (resistance) to the exercise being done.

The goal of a good strengthening program is to "overload" your muscles just enough to get them to adapt to the extra work by becoming stronger. This can be done by adding hand-held or wrap-around weights, elastic bands or simply by using the weight of your body. Avoid loading muscles so much that they are sore and stiff for a day or two after exercising.

If you have active inflammation, or if you feel you need to protect certain joints, check with a therapist about which strengthening exercises are best and safest for you. If you have been inactive, start by doing 15 minutes of flexibility exercises before you attempt any strengthening ones.

CARDIOVASCULAR (AEROBIC) EXERCISES

When you hear "aerobics," do you think of young adults in skimpy clothes working up a sweat while loud music blares? Aerobic exercise means more than just aerobic dance. Also known as cardiovascular or endurance exercise, aerobic exercise is any physical activity that uses the large muscles of the body in rhythmic, continuous motions. Walking, dancing, swimming, bicycling or even raking leaves are all examples of aerobic exercise.

These exercises make up the third important part of your exercise routine. The pur-

Finding Your Target Heart Rate

To find your target heart rate, you must stop during your activity and take your pulse. Keep walking or moving around to keep your blood circulating. Placing your index and middle fingers on your opposite wrist or below your jawline at your neck, count your pulse for six seconds and add a zero to that number (or count for 10 seconds and multiply by six). For example, if you count 14 beats in a 10-second period, your heart rate is six times 14, or 84 beats per minute.

Using the chart for a guide, find the target heart rate for your age group. You don't want your heart rate to be faster than the top end of the range during your aerobic exercise. If it does exceed the maximum, slow it down! If you are a beginner, consider the higher number in your range as a "not-to-exceed" heart rate. And take heart: If you exercise in your target range regularly, your endurance and conditioning will improve.

pose of aerobic exercise is to make your heart, lungs, blood vessels and muscles work more efficiently. This general involvement of the body promotes overall health by reducing your risk of heart disease, high blood pressure and diabetes. For people with arthritis, aerobic exercise can help improve endurance, strengthen bones, improve sleep, control weight, and reduce depression and anxiety.

Your fitness program should include some aerobic activities three to four times each week. The goal is to work within your target heart rate for 30 minutes each session. If you are not able to exercise continuously for

30 minutes, work up to it slowly. Start with five minutes of gradually increasing activity, continue with five minutes of activity in your recommended heart range (see p.146), then decrease activity for five minutes. Once you are able to do this, you can increase the length of activity in your target range.

Walking. Walking is an excellent type of aerobic exercise for almost everyone. It requires no special skills and is inexpensive. You will need a good pair of supportive walking shoes, and you may need orthotics or special shoe inserts. You can walk almost anytime and anywhere. Many towns now have mall walking clubs, providing a safe place to exercise whatever the weather outside.

Water exercise. Swimming and exercising in warm water are especially good for stiff joints and sore muscles. Water helps support your body while you move your joints through their range of motion. Swimming is highly recommended as an aerobic workout, because little stress is placed on your joints.

Bicycling. Cycling on a stationary bicycle is a good way to get aerobic exercise without placing much stress on your hips, knees or feet. Some stationary bicycles allow you to exercise your upper body as well. When beginning, try not to pedal faster than 15 to 20 miles per hour. As you become more fit you can increase your speed and/or add resistance to your workout.

Rowing. Rowing on a machine – or if you are lucky enough, in a boat – is a good aerobic exercise for people with hip, knee or foot involvement.

Ski machines. Cross-country skiing or using a machine that simulates that action is an excellent nonimpact exercise. It is one of the least abrasive non-water exercises and it works both the upper and lower body.

A Note About Pain

You may be afraid to exercise too vigorously for fear of causing pain or damage to your joints. This is a common concern for many people with rheumatoid arthritis. It is important to recognize that gentle exercise is best. You can learn to tell the difference between the type of pain you experience from sore muscles after exercising, and the type of pain caused by overuse or inflammation of joints.

Sore muscles are usually the result of overstretching muscles or overusing them when you have been inactive. This type of pain usually begins several hours after exercising and may continue for 24 to 36 hours.

If you experience muscle soreness, you may try spending more time doing flexibility or warm-up exercises before proceeding to more vigorous activity. You may want to scale back your program until your muscles become more accustomed to a certain level of exercise, then gradually increase your workout.

By contrast, swelling and pain may be a signal of overuse of joints. If you notice these symptoms, you can treat the joint by elevating and resting it. You may need to modify your exercise program to avoid further stress to the joint.

One further note about pain: Exercise has been found to be one of the most consistently effective nondrug tools you can use to reduce the pain associated with arthritis. So exercise sensibly, but do exercise. You *will* feel better.

Don't Go It Alone

Many people who exercise on their own find it hard to stay motivated and keep going. If you are among these people, it may help to exercise with at least one other person. Two or more people can keep each other motivated, while joining a class can give you a feeling of shared goals and camaraderie.

Most communities offer a variety of exercise classes, including special programs for people with arthritis, people over 50 or those who need adaptive exercises. The Arthritis Foundation sponsors exercise programs taught by trained instructors and developed specifically for people with arthritis. For information, contact your local chapter or branch office. Programs are also available through local YMCA organizations, health clubs, hospital-sponsored fitness facilities, community colleges, parks and recreation departments, and senior centers.

If you would like to join a community exercise class or health club, try to find one

Personally Speaking Stories from real people with rheumatoid arthritis

"As I sat in the New Orleans airport waiting for my sister to arrive, my heart was pounding. She had been diagnosed with rheumatoid arthritis two months before. The occasion of her visit was her 40th birthday, and I wanted this to be a joyous celebration. But I found myself feeling tearful as I waited for her plane to land. When I saw her, I breathed a sigh of relief. She didn't look any different, just slightly more somber.

Rheumatoid Arthritis From the Outside: A Sister's View
by Beth Hodgens, Macon, GA

"This was five years ago. I was fortunate enough to celebrate my sister's 45th birthday just recently. She came to my hometown to play in a regional tennis championship. She and her partner blew their opponents away in the final match of the weekend.

"My sister is a single parent of two teenage boys, and the director of marketing at a large hospital in Atlanta. Her motto has always been 'Keep moving.' Since her diagnosis with rheumatoid arthritis, there is new meaning in that phrase. Her ability to keep all the balls in the air, her attitude and her movement have helped her gain a handle on her disease. She is a hero to me!"

offering classes that meet your needs. Try to find staff members who are certified by a professional organization, with training or experience in teaching exercise for people with arthritis or other special needs. The facilities, including the bathroom and changing areas, should be physically accessible. In addition, you should feel at ease and comfortable with the staff and other members. Let your instructors know your concerns about special needs or modifications. If a facility does not offer you what you need, or you don't feel comfortable exercising there, you may wish to find another one. If you don't enjoy exercising, you probably won't stick with it.

Sample Exercises

Here are some sample flexibility and strengthening exercises that you can use in either a warm-up or a cool-down. Note the precautions, if any, and select the exercises that are best for you. You might check with your doctor first before beginning a new exercise program or routine if you are concerned. But most of the time, you are the best person to decide what exercises are best for you. All these exercises are acceptable for some people with rheumatoid arthritis but all are not appropriate for *all* people with rheumatoid arthritis. Use common sense and check with your doctor or therapist if you're not sure.

NECK EXERCISES

Purpose. Increase neck movement. Relax tense neck and shoulder muscles. Improve posture.

Precautions. Do slowly and smoothly. If you feel dizzy, stop the exercise. If you have had neck problems, check with your doctor or therapist before doing these exercises.

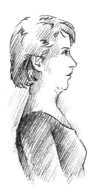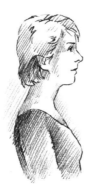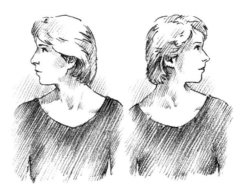

I. CHIN TUCKS
Pull your chin back as if to make a double chin. Keep your head straight – don't look down. Hold three seconds. Then raise your neck straight up as if someone was pulling straight up on your hair.

2. HEAD TURNS (ROTATION)
Turn your head to look over your shoulder. Hold three seconds. Return to the center and then turn to look over your other shoulder. Hold three seconds. Repeat.

SHOULDER GIRDLE EXERCISES

Purpose. Increase mobility of the shoulder girdle (the bony structure that supports your upper limbs). Strengthen muscles that raise shoulders. Relax tense neck and shoulder muscles.

Precautions. If the exercise increases pain, discontinue and consult your doctor.

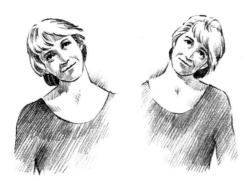

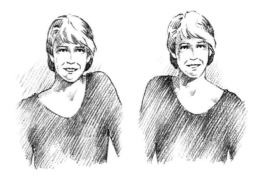

3. HEAD TILTS

Focus on an object in front of you. Tilt your head sideways toward your right shoulder. Hold three seconds. Return to the center and tilt toward your left shoulder. Hold three seconds. Do not twist head but continue to look forward. Do not raise your shoulder toward your ear.

4. SHOULDER SHRUGS (ELEVATION)

(A) Raise one shoulder, lower it. Then raise the other shoulder. Be sure the first shoulder is completely relaxed and lowered before raising the other. (B) Raise both shoulders up toward the ears. Hold three seconds. Relax. Concentrate on completely relaxing shoulders as they come down. Do not tilt the head or body in either direction. Do not hunch shoulders forward or pinch shoulder blades together.

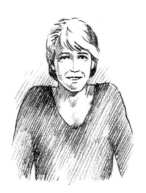

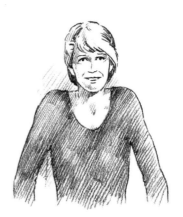

5. SHOULDER CIRCLES

Lift both shoulders up, move them forward, then down and back in a circling motion. Then lift both shoulders up, move them backward, then down and forward in a circling motion.

ARM EXERCISES (SHOULDERS AND ELBOWS)

Purpose. Increase shoulder and/or elbow motion. Strengthen shoulder and/or elbow muscles. Relax tense neck and shoulder muscles. Improve posture.

Precautions. If you have had shoulder or elbow surgery, check with your surgeon before doing these exercises. These exercises are not advised for people with significant shoulder joint damage, such as unstable joints or total cuff tears.

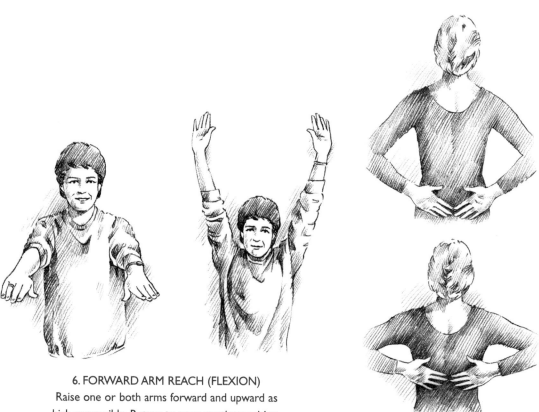

6. FORWARD ARM REACH (FLEXION)
Raise one or both arms forward and upward as high as possible. Return to your starting position.

7. SELF BACK RUB (INTERNAL ROTATION)
While seated, slide a few inches forward from the back of your chair. Sit up as straight as possible, do not round your shoulders. Place the back of your hands on your lower back. Slowly move them upward until you feel a stretch in your shoulders. Hold three seconds, then slide your hands back down. You can use one hand to help the other. Move within the limits of your pain. Do not force.

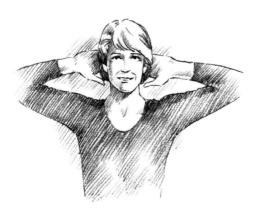 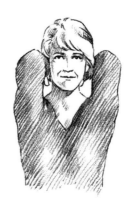

8. SHOULDER ROTATOR

Sit or stand as straight as possible. Reach up and place your hands on the back of your head. (If you cannot reach your head, place your arms in a "muscle man" position with elbows bent in a right angle and upper arm at shoulder level.) Take a deep breath in. As you breathe out, bring your elbows together in front of you. Slowly move elbows apart as you breathe in.

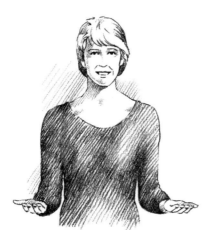 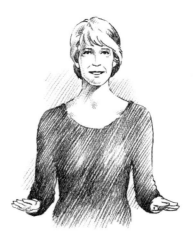

9. DOOR OPENER (PRONATION AND SUPINATION)

Bend your elbows and hold them in to your sides. Your forearms should be parallel to the floor. Slowly turn forearms and palms to face the ceiling. Hold three seconds and then turn them slowly toward the floor.

WRIST EXERCISES

Purpose. Increase wrist motion. Strengthen wrist muscles.

Precaution. If you have had wrist or elbow surgery, check with your doctor before doing this exercise. Stop if you feel any numbness or tingling.

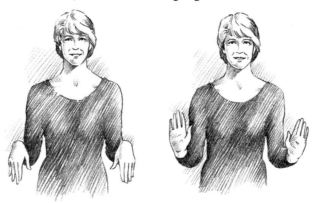

10. WRIST BEND (EXTENSION)

If sitting, rest hands and forearms on thighs, table, or arms of chair. If standing, bend your elbows and hold hands in front of you, palms down. Lift up palms and fingers, keeping forearms flat. Hold three seconds. Relax.

FINGER EXERCISES

Purpose. Increase finger motion. Increase ability to grip and hold objects.

Precautions. If the exercise increases finger pain, stop and consult your doctor.

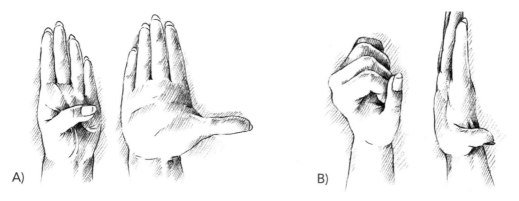

A)

B)

11. THUMB BEND AND FINGER CURL (FLEXION/EXTENSION)

(A) With hands open and fingers relaxed, reach thumb across your palm and try to touch the base of your little finger. Hold three seconds. Stretch thumb back out to the other side as far as possible.

(B) Make a loose fist by curling all your fingers into your palm. Keep your thumb out. Hold for three seconds. Then stretch out your fingers to straighten them.

TRUNK EXERCISES

Purpose. Increase trunk flexibility. Stretch and strengthen back and abdominal muscles.

Precautions. If you have osteoporosis, back compression fracture, previous back surgery or a hip replacement, check with your doctor before doing these exercises. Do not bend your body forward or backward unless specifically told to do so. Move slowly and immediately stop any exercise that causes you back or neck pain.

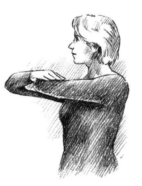

12. SIDE BENDS

While standing, keep weight evenly on both hips. Lean toward the right and reach your fingers toward the floor. Hold three seconds. Return to center and repeat exercise toward the left. Do not lean forward or backward while bending, and do not twist the torso.

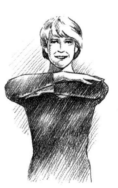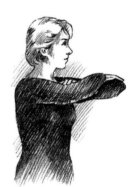

13. TRUNK TWIST (ROTATION)

Place your hands on your hips, straight out to the side, crossed over your chest, or on opposite elbows. Twist your body around to look over your right shoulder. Hold three seconds. Return to the center and then twist to the left. Be sure you are twisting at the waist and not at your neck or hips. NOTE: Vary the exercise by holding a ball in front of or next to your body.

LOWER BODY EXERCISES

Purpose. Increase lower body strength. Increase range of motion in hip, knee and ankle joints.

Precautions. Check with your surgeon before doing these exercises if you have had hip, knee, ankle, foot or toe surgery or any lower extremity joint replacement. Do not rotate the upper body unless specifically told to do so.

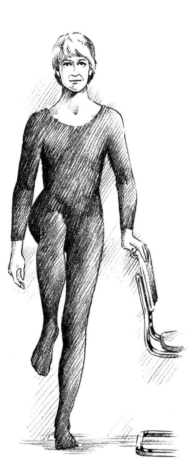

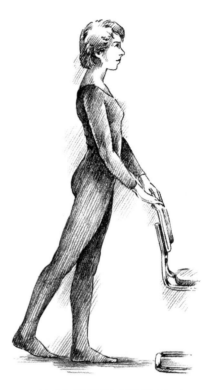

15. BACK KICK (HIP EXTENSION)

Stand straight on one leg and lift the other leg behind you. Hold three seconds. Try to keep your leg straight as you move it backward. Motion should occur only in the hip (not waist). Do not lean forward – keep your upper body straight. NOTE: You can add resistance by using a large rubber exercise band around ankles.

14. MARCH (HIP/KNEE FLEXION)

Stand sideways to a chair and lightly grasp the back. If you feel unsteady, hold onto two chairs or face the back of the chair. Alternate lifting your legs up and down as if marching in place. Gradually try to lift knees higher and/or march faster.

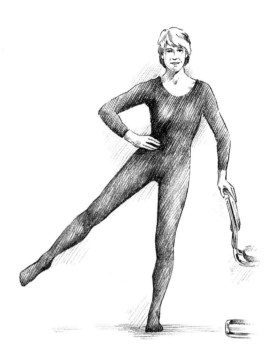

16. SIDE LEG KICK
(HIP ABDUCTION/ADDUCTION)

Stand near a chair, holding it for support. Stand on one leg and lift the other leg out to the side. Hold three seconds and return your leg to the floor. Only move your leg at the top – don't lean toward the chair. Alternate legs.

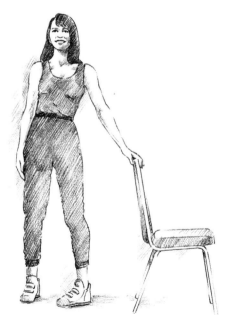

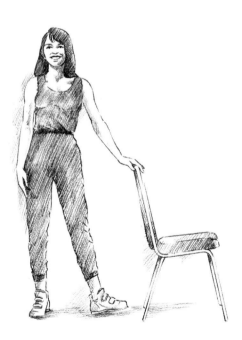

17. HIP TURNS (INTERNAL/EXTERNAL ROTATION)

Stand with legs slightly apart, with your weight on one leg and the heel of your other foot lightly touching the floor. Rotate your whole leg from the hip so that toes and knee point in and then out. Don't rotate your body – keep chest and shoulders facing forward. NOTE: If you have difficulty putting weight on one leg, you can also do this exercise by sitting at the edge of a chair with your legs extended straight in front and with your heels resting on the floor.

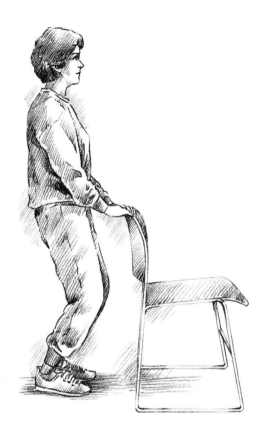

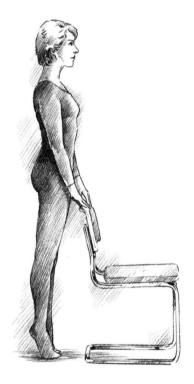

18. SKIER'S SQUAT (QUADRICEPS STRENGTHENER)
Stand behind a chair with your hands lightly resting on top of chair for support. Keep your feet flat on the floor. Keeping your back straight, slowly bend your knees to lower your body a few inches. Hold for three to six seconds, then slowly return to an upright position.

19. TIPTOE (DORSI/PLANTAR FLEXION)
Face the back of a chair and rest your hands on it. Rise up and stand on your toes. Hold three seconds, then return to the flat position. Try to keep your knees straight (but not locked). Now stand on your heels, raising your toes and front part of your foot off the ground. NOTE: You can do this exercise one foot at a time.

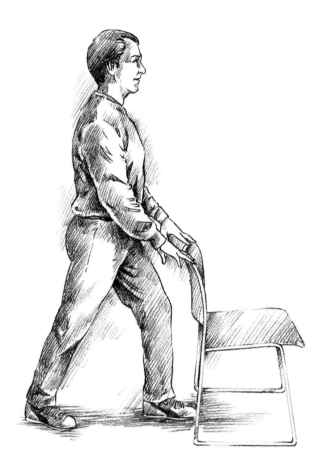

20. CALF STRETCH (GASTROC-SOLEUS STRETCH)
Hold lightly to the back of a chair. Bend the knee of the leg you are not stretching
so that it almost touches the chair. Put the leg to be stretched behind you, keeping
both feet flat on the floor. Lean forward gently, keeping your back knee straight.

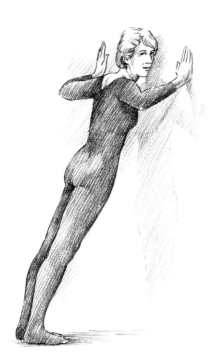

21. CHEST STRETCH
(HIP EXTENSION AND PECTORALIS STRETCH)

Stand about two to three feet away from a wall and place your hands or forearms on the wall at shoulder height. Lean forward, leading with your hips. Keep your knees straight and your head back. Hold this position for five to 10 seconds, then push back to starting position. To feel more stretch, place your hands farther apart.

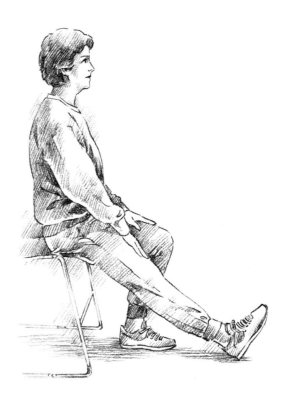

22. THIGH FIRMER AND KNEE STRETCH

Sit on the edge of your chair or lie on your back with your legs stretched out in front and your heels resting on the floor. Tighten the muscle that runs across the front of the knee by pulling your toes toward your head. Push the back of the knee down toward the floor so you also feel a stretch at the back of your knee and ankle. For a greater stretch, put your heel on a footstool and lean forward as you pull your toes toward your head.

Chapter 16

When You Feel Exhausted:

Coping With Fatigue

Fatigue is one of the most common symptoms experienced by people with rheumatoid arthritis. Sometimes it is the first sign of inflammation. During periods of inflammatory activity, it is not unusual for people to feel overwhelmingly fatigued, with no energy at all. This overwhelming fatigue can impair your ability to concentrate, make you less able to deal with pain, and increase your feelings of helplessness. Like pain, fatigue is a signal that something is wrong. It is important to pay attention to this signal.

Fatigue may be caused by several different factors including inflammation of rheumatoid arthritis, overdoing routine activities, medication side effects, stress and depression. A lack of restful sleep, poor nutrition and absence of regular exercise also may increase feelings of fatigue.

Feeling tired all the time can lead to a nonproductive cycle of more stress and depression, leaving you less able to meet daily challenges. And, if you become physically run-down, your immune system becomes less resistant to infection and illness. In this chapter, we will provide some tools to help you decipher the causes of your fatigue and strategies for managing it. Although some fatigue may be unavoidable, you can eliminate certain sources and triggers of fatigue by being a good self-manager. By setting priorities, making smart choices and conserving your strength, you will still be able to do most of what is important to you.

Pinpointing Causes of Your Fatigue

Your fatigue may be caused by physical, emotional and environmental factors. The box on page 162 lists some of the more common physical and emotional causes of fatigue, and lists some actions that you can take to address them. In addition to these, environmental factors such as high noise levels, temperature variations, and even daily hassles such as dealing with traffic and waiting in line, can make you feel tired.

Identifying the Causes of Your Fatigue

PHYSICAL CAUSES

Are you experiencing a flare of rheumatoid arthritis? The process of inflammation can make you feel tired all over.

Action: Discuss a possible change in your treatment plan, such as increasing dosages of medication to control the flare.

Are you overdoing activities or pushing yourself too hard? Fatigue can be a signal that you are doing too much.

Action: Cut down on the number of tasks you do each day. Learn to alternate periods of activity with breaks.

Have you been doing very little? Too much inactivity leads to muscle deconditioning and can actually make you feel worse.

Action: Incorporate more physical activity into your daily routine (see chapter 15). A therapist can show you safe and gentle exercises that won't harm your joints.

Are you taking any new medications? Fatigue can be a side effect of some medications.

Action: Talk to your doctor or pharmacist about your concerns. It may be possible to switch medications or take them at different times during the day.

Do you awaken feeling rested? If not, you may have insomnia caused by pain.

Action: Your doctor or pharmacist may suggest medications that can ease your pain or help you sleep. Also see tips on getting a good night's sleep in this chapter.

Is your fatigue accompanied by all-over muscle pain or tenderness? If so, you may have fibromyalgia in addition to your arthritis.

Action: Describe your symptoms to your doctor. He or she may prescribe an additional medication, or provide exercise or relaxation tips.

EMOTIONAL CAUSES

Are you experiencing more stress than usual? Your body's response to stress uses up energy, particularly if stress is continuous.

Action: Track your stress using a diary, as discussed in Chapter 13. Prioritize your tasks to conserve energy.

Have you been worrying more lately? It's natural to have worries and concerns, particularly when you have a chronic disease. However, worry drains energy and can become a compulsive habit.

Action: Try using relaxation techniques or sharing your concerns with your spouse or a friend. Write down your worries and then try to find solutions.

Do you feel depressed? People who have clinical depression often experience fatigue.

Action: Seek professional help if you think you may have symptoms of depression. Also, read Chapter 13 for information on dealing with depression.

USING A FATIGUE WORKSHEET

One way to help you discover the causes of your fatigue is to use a fatigue diary similar to the one shown below. In it, you can note the times of the day or week when you feel fatigue and also what seems to trigger the feeling. Although it may seem like a lot of work, sometimes it's possible to see an obvious solution to the problem that you might otherwise miss. For instance, people often blame themselves for overdoing it when they feel tired, but by reviewing your fatigue sheet you may see that your fatigue is actually a sign of increased disease activity that calls for a change in your treatment plan. You may wish to discuss this with your doctor.

Fatigue Problem-Solving Worksheet

CAUSE OF FATIGUE	POSSIBLE SOLUTIONS

What Your Doctor Can Do

When fatigue is due to inflammation, it is often more easily corrected than when it is due to stress. The inflammatory *cytokines* (protein molecules) that are released in rheumatoid arthritis are the same chemicals that are released when you have a severe cold or flu. Although in rheumatoid arthritis they are not fighting to protect your body from disease, they can still leave you feeling weak and tired. Your doctor can improve this type of fatigue by prescribing higher doses of your current drugs or another drug to be used alone or in combination to control the body's inflammatory process. Once inflammation is under control, fatigue usually lessens.

It is also important to consider other potential sources of fatigue that your doctor can reverse. One possibility is *anemia*, which occurs when the body has too few red blood cells to effectively transport oxygen. A particular type of anemia, often called "the anemia of chronic disease" is often seen in people with rheumatoid arthritis. Effective treatment of arthritis often resolves this type of anemia. Another cause of anemia is due to blood loss from stomach ulcers, and this may require iron replacement and other treatments.

Another consideration is whether the medications themselves are causing fatigue. Fatigue is a side effect of many medications — not usually the drugs used to treat rheumatoid arthritis, but drugs for other conditions such as hypertension (high blood pressure) or depression. Ask your doctor if any medications you are taking cause fatigue, and

whether any adjustments can be made to improve the situation. Fibromyalgia (see Chapter 5) is also common in people with rheumatoid arthritis, and may cause fatigue.

If you have a second chronic condition (that is, a medical condition in addition to rheumatoid arthritis), your level of fatigue may be even higher. For instance, people with thyroid disease or lung problems often feel fatigued for reasons other than inflammation. If you and your doctor address these additional problems, your level of energy should increase.

Sometimes fatigue can be aggravated by not being able to get a good night's sleep. While we will discuss some ways that you can improve your sleep habits, another option is the use of sleeping pills. In some situations, pills to promote sleep can be of great advantage for people with rheumatoid arthritis. Some people have a very good experience with sleeping pills, but others find they don't work well for them. You can work with your doctor to determine the best approach to the use of sleeping pills and which ones might work best for you.

What You Can Do

The most effective approach you can take when dealing with fatigue is to be aware that it is a part of rheumatoid arthritis, and that you might have to adapt your schedule to fatigue, rather than fight it. Don't consider fatigue a sign of personal weakness or deny it. It is simply one more symptom of arthritis that you can learn to handle.

For example, many people with rheumatoid arthritis adjust their daily schedule to start one or two hours later. This delay in starting the day makes it easier to deal with morning stiffness and may also enable you to sleep longer.

Ultimately, the result is less fatigue and a more productive day. Other people may take a rest or nap in the afternoon, which then allows them to continue with their daily activities without collapsing from fatigue at the end of the day.

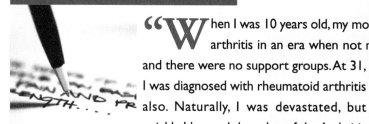

Personally Speaking — Stories from real people with rheumatoid arthritis

"When I was 10 years old, my mother was diagnosed with rheumatoid arthritis in an era when not much was known about the disease, and there were no support groups. At 31, I was diagnosed with rheumatoid arthritis also. Naturally, I was devastated, but quickly I learned the value of the Arthritis Foundation and its wealth of guidance and educational material.

My Nine Self-Management Guidelines
by Karen Lenker
Berwyn, PA

"The first step was to choose a physician, one I had good rapport with, for I knew the doctor would be a major part of my life and my friend. I have learned a lot of emotional coping and self-management skills from others. Hopefully, these skills will help someone else, like other people have helped me over the years. They are:

1. Before my feet hit the ground in the morning, I think of 10 things to be grateful for.

2. Exercise in the morning, either walking, riding a stationary bike, or doing exercises or water aerobics at the YMCA.

3. Take time dressing and grooming. Nice soap, cologne, attention to jewelry, or a scarf can perk you up. Most major stores have personal shoppers, and this service can save you lots of energy.

4. Schedule ahead so your days aren't so busy. Include time for rest.

5. Make lists to save time. I always keep a small notepad with me. Doctor's appointments are more productive with a list of subjects to be addressed.

6. Educate family and friends about your arthritis verbally, or with printed material from the Arthritis Foundation.

7. Ask for help ahead of time, so others can put you in their schedules. Sometimes I give a family member a written list to eliminate constant asking.

8. Have fun! Church, hobbies, movies and reading will keep you connected with other people. Support groups are invaluable.

9. Do something for someone else. Help someone in need with an errand, visit or listening ear. Correspond with an old friend or relative. Volunteer."

Using a fatigue diary can help you determine when you feel most tired, and help you adjust your schedule accordingly. Is it right after a heavy lunch? Or do you get sleepy after working at the computer all morning? Try varying your tasks and taking brief breaks to stretch and move around. If you are able, plan to take a walk during your lunch hour a few days a week. Avoid eating heavy meals; instead, opt for a light lunch, perhaps with a healthy morning and afternoon snack thrown in.

Rest is crucial, but it's not the only game in town. It is also important to recognize that doing too little can often lead to deconditioning – which in turn makes you feel more fatigued. Moderate exercise keeps your muscles and joints in condition, and has the added benefit of helping you sleep better at night. There is validity to the conventional wisdom that you get energy by using it!

UNDERSTANDING YOUR BODY'S RHYTHMS

Recent research has shown that people have natural tendencies to be most awake at certain hours and most rested at other hours. These patterns are referred to as your body's *circadian rhythms*. Most people seem to be "morning people" and have their most alert hours in the morning, tend to go to sleep by 9 p.m. to 11 p.m., sleep for seven to eight hours, and awaken between 6 a.m. and 7 a.m. However, some people are "night people" who find it difficult to get up in the morning and feel tired all day if they are forced to get up before restful sleep can occur.

For years, scientists believed that people could change their body's natural rhythms over time, but new findings suggest these adjustments are more complex than first thought. A night person who has to rise before 6 a.m. may often feel fatigued all day, unless a nap is possible. Study your own body's natural rhythms, and you may be able to determine the best time to go to sleep and to wake up. Of course, it is impossible to plan your daily schedule completely, but the more you can be in harmony with your natural rhythms, the less likely you will suffer from a high level of fatigue.

GETTING A GOOD NIGHT'S SLEEP

A lack of restful sleep is a problem shared by a great many Americans, and can be due to many different factors. These may include stress; depression; use of caffeine, alcohol or drugs; not allowing enough time for sleep; and pain. When you have rheumatoid arthritis, pain may keep you from falling asleep easily, or it may awaken you during the night. Research has shown that some people with rheumatoid arthritis experience light, easily disrupted sleep with many mid-sleep awakenings. This leads to higher levels of fatigue.

There are several stages of sleep. During the night, your brain moves between these stages in cycles, and the types of electrical brain waves generated vary from stage to stage. To really feel rested, your brain requires what is called "delta sleep," named after the brain waves that occur in the third and fourth stages of sleep. REM (short for rapid eye movement) sleep is also important. It's the stage of sleep when dreaming occurs, and missing it can leave you feeling tired in the morning.

Aging and menopause cause changes in sleep patterns. As people age, there is an increasing variability in the amount and quality of sleep. In older individuals, there is a tendency to spend less time in deep (restorative) sleep and to sleep for shorter periods. Menopause, which usually occurs in the late 40s through early 50s for women, can also cause sleep disturbances such as hot flashes and frequent awakening during the night. Hormone replacement therapy may help alleviate these symptoms.

So, how can you get the sleep you need? Review the checklist on this page for some helpful suggestions, but be aware that it may take time to change your ingrained patterns. If you feel anxious about getting to sleep, you might consider adding some relaxation exercises to your nighttime routine as well.

PRIORITIZING YOUR TIME AND ENERGY

There may be times when you feel more fatigued than others, and you will have to deal with limitations to your energy. Think of your energy as a resource that you have to conserve to have enough for the most important activities. This may involve saying no to lower priority activities that take up too much of your energy.

Checklist for Getting the Sleep You Need

Establish Regular Sleep Patterns
- Try to go to bed and arise at the same time each day.
- Avoid taking naps too close to bedtime.
- Take a warm to hot bath within two hours of bedtime.
- A warm, non-caffeinated drink may help you relax.

Create a Restful Environment
- Make sure your bedroom is dark, quiet and comfortable.
- Avoid bright light if you have to arise during the sleep period.
- Keep your clock turned away from you.

Exercise
- Exercise regularly each day.
- Avoid vigorous exercise or activity for at least two hours prior to bedtime.

Be Aware of Drug Effects
- Give up smoking, or avoid smoking several hours before bedtime.
- Limit use of alcoholic beverages.
- Cut back or discontinue drinking caffeinated beverages.
- Use prescribed sleep medication only as directed.

Other Considerations
- Avoid large meals two to three hours before bedtime.
- Menopause and aging may cause changes to your established sleep patterns.
- If pain keeps you from sleeping, discuss medication options with your doctor.

Reprinted from *Clinical Care in the Rheumatic Diseases*. Used with permission of the American College of Rheumatology.

Of course, it's not always easy to say no, but it helps to stay focused on the priorities in your life, such as earning a living or spending time with your children. When you're feeling fatigued, opting out of an activity may allow you to get the rest you need at this time. Saying no to one activity may allow you to say yes to something more important to you at a later time. Chapter 14 may provide some additional ideas on ways to prioritize your activities and conserve your energy.

ASK FOR HELP, EVEN IF IT'S DIFFICULT

Successful managers are people who have learned that they cannot do everything themselves. Borrowing from their techniques, you can learn to delegate the tasks of managing your activities. Asking for help may be difficult at first. Because the effects of rheumatoid arthritis are not always visible to the outside observer, you may be afraid that co-workers and acquaintances will perceive you as lazy.

You may feel embarrassed to ask for help, especially if you've always prided yourself on being a high achiever. The following suggestions can make it easier to request help from others:

- **Ask for specific help.** For example, if you ask someone to take you shopping for one hour every other Tuesday morning, you are letting them know precisely the help you need. Also, you show others that you understand their time is valuable as well.
- **Develop a "pool" of helpers.** Spreading out the load of additional tasks keeps the burden from falling on any one person. Keep a list of friends and family and which tasks they're willing to help with.
- **Consider bartering or trading services with others.** If you dislike asking for help, perhaps you can provide a service in return. For instance, you can offer to watch your friend's children one afternoon a week at your house, if she will run some errands for you.

Chapter 17

Pushing
the Boundaries:

Complementary and Alternative Therapies

One of several messages we hope you have gotten from this book is that there are no easy answers for the complex problems caused by rheumatoid arthritis. Rheumatoid arthritis affects each person individually, making treatment decisions sometimes seem arbitrary. Standard or conventional medicine has no "cures" for arthritis, as it does for infections, stomach ulcers and other diseases.

Because of these reasons, the issue of complementary and alternative therapies has always been a sort of subtext to the treatment program. Study after study has shown that people with arthritis do turn to these therapies, in part due to the fact that drugs do not control disease symptoms completely, and also due to patients' dissatisfaction with the present system of health care. In fact, a 1998 study reported that nearly half of all Americans are trying some kind of unconventional, alternative or complementary therapy.

According to most definitions, an *alternative therapy* is any practice or substance outside the realm of conventional medicine. *Complementary therapy* includes practices that coexist with traditional treatment. Many of these complementary therapies, such as exercise and relaxation, have already been discussed in earlier chapters of this book. Here, our focus will be on some of the more unconventional ones, which are truly "alternative."

Alternative therapies can provide a sense of self-direction and control to people who have chronic health conditions. Some of these treatments, however, fly in the face of accepted scientific principles and natural laws. When accompanied by aggressive or misleading marketing tactics that promise a "cure" for arthritis, many doctors in the past tended to react negatively and refused to discuss these therapies with their patients.

With the establishment in 1992 of the National Institutes of Health Office of

Alternative Medicine, now known as the National Center for Complementary and Alternative Medicine (NCCAM), alternative therapies have come out of the closet, so to speak. Many health-care providers realize their patients may try these unconventional remedies and that it is better to discuss such alternatives – and their potential effects – with patients than to ignore the issue.

It would be impossible to discuss the many dozens (perhaps hundreds) of complementary and alternative therapies in a single chapter. Our goal will be to discuss some broad categories of unconventional therapies, then give you information that can help you discuss this topic with your doctor, as well as help you make informed choices about these treatments.

The Arthritis Foundation has published a book, *The Arthritis Foundation's Guide to Alternative Therapies*, filled with information on this topic, if you would like more in-depth information about individual therapies.

Types of Complementary and Alternative Therapy

(Note to reader: Relaxation and stress reduction techniques, such as guided imagery and relaxation exercises are discussed in Chapter 13. Exercise is covered in Chapter 15. Although considered complementary therapies, they are recognized as an important part of a comprehensive arthritis management program.)

MASSAGE

Massage therapy is considered by many health professionals to be an excellent way of easing the pain and stiffness associated with arthritis. It can help stretch tight muscles, improve flexibility, and ease pain and stress. Massage is usually categorized as a complementary therapy; in fact, rheumatologists often recommend massage for arthritis and related conditions. Evidence from scientific studies has shown that massage can decrease stress hormones and depression, ease muscle pain and spasms, increase the body's production of natural pain-killing endorphins, and improve sleep and immune function.

Although many different types of massage are available, most include a combination of strokes, friction and pressure that are used to help relax the muscles. Some types, such as Swedish massage, emphasize the physical by using pressing, rubbing and manipulation to work on muscles and joints to improve function. Asian techniques emphasize balancing the flow of vital energy in your body. There are even some techniques – such as reiki and therapeutic touch – that focus on energy for spiritual healing, and practitioners don't physically touch you at all.

What can you expect from your massage? Your session may be given on a padded table or a mat on the floor in a warm, quiet room. It may be softly lit, with quiet music, or it may be more like a typical doctor's office. Before starting, the therapist may talk to you about any special health conditions or sensitivities (such as actively inflamed or painful joints), and discuss your goals for the session. You do not have to remove all of your clothes; often, the therapist will cover you with a large sheet and will uncover only the part of your body that is being massaged.

Sessions vary in length from about 45 minutes to an hour and a half, and cost from $50 to $100 per hour (although prices vary by location and expertise of the therapist). During that time, the therapist will periodically ask how you are or tell you what to do. You should speak up at any time if you feel pain or discomfort, or if you have questions. After the session, most people feel relaxed but energized. Any soreness you feel from the massage should disappear by the next day. If it does not, discuss it with your therapist before the next session.

Although massage is beneficial for many people, it is best to use caution before seeking out a therapist. Therapists may not have experience in participating in the care of people with rheumatoid arthritis, and may not understand their physical needs. Some

Personally Speaking Stories from real people with rheumatoid arthritis

"'Energy begets energy' used to be my mantra. 'Movement is life!' my message resounded. Now, the swelling in my joints tells me the truth. Movement is a *gift*.

"I want to exercise. I am sick and tired of my excuses for not being able to participate. Why can't I be the old, energy-packed me? Sure, my excuses are real. I am in my fifth year of rheumatoid arthritis. I have tried to cope with it and accept it. The flares are crippling and strike with no apparent reason. One day I am feeling well, the next day I have hot liquid burning in my joints. Cortisone injections punctured into the offending joints are my only relief.

The Other Side Of Fitness
by Meredith Bunting, Virginia Beach, VA

"I walk with swollen, cramped feet to greet members in the health club I have managed for 10 years. I direct them to the exercise equipment, and tell them about various energy-packed fitness classes — the ones I used to teach. As they press on to chosen activities, I slip back behind my wall of memories.

"On their way to exercise, my friends greet me. Their smiles touch me like rays of sunshine dispersing murky clouds. They treat me as if nothing has changed. Oh, they know I have had a 'setback.' But they believe in me. They don't pity me. They offer help and lend a hand. I begin to see another side of fitness. It is compassion in action.

"As I accept their help, I sense my walls crumbling. Letting go of what I can no longer do, and inspired by the helping spirit of my friends, I feel a new source of energy. This side of fitness has great potential!"

elements of massage may not be appropriate for people with rheumatoid arthritis. It is best not to have an inflamed joint massaged; in fact, it may make the joint feel worse. Finally, be aware that massage may not be covered by your insurance policy, even when suggested by your doctor.

ACUPUNCTURE/ACUPRESSURE

Long a cornerstone of Chinese medicine, *acupuncture* has been making its way to the Western world for the treatment of many chronic conditions, including arthritis. In acupuncture, disposable stainless steel needles are used to stimulate specific points – located in energy pathways called *meridians* – throughout the body. These pathways have no counterpart in conventional medicine and anatomy.

More than 15 million Americans have used acupuncture, primarily for pain relief. Acupuncture has been used to treat many kinds of arthritis, including rheumatoid arthritis. Some studies have suggested that acupuncture may lessen pain by causing the body to release *endorphins* (naturally produced chemicals that block pain messages and prevent them from reaching the brain). There have also been suggestions that acupuncture has anti-inflammatory effects, but further research is needed to document these phenomena. You are the best judge of whether or not acupuncture is helpful to you.

Acupuncture sessions usually last from 30 minutes to one hour (longer on your first visit) and may cost up to $75 per session. You will be asked to sit or lie on a padded table, to remove or loosen clothing, and to get comfortable before treatment starts. A traditional practitioner of Chinese acupuncture may ask you many questions about your health, diet and sleep habits. For the treatment itself, the practitioner will use from two to 15 thin needles, which are inserted at specific points that relate to your condition in Chinese medicine. This treatment may be combined with heat or electrical stimulation.

You should not feel pain, although you may experience slight discomfort when the needles are inserted. The acupuncturist will leave you resting with the needles in place for a short period (20 minutes is typical). Once the needles are removed, you will rest quietly for a while before getting up.

Although the World Health Organization has endorsed the use of acupuncture to treat rheumatoid arthritis, many studies have failed to document the effectiveness of this therapy. If you decide to try acupuncture, find a practitioner who is certified or licensed. Some health insurers will cover these treatments if they are prescribed by (or performed by) a doctor. In addition, make sure that the practitioner uses only sterile, disposable needles.

The idea of having someone insert needles into your body may not seem appealing to everyone. Many people get some of the same benefits from *acupressure*, which is an even older form of this therapy. Instead of needles, practitioners use their fingers or other tools to apply pressure to the same points used in acupuncture.

SPECIAL DIETS OR DIETARY CHANGES

The myth of the miracle arthritis diet is one of the oldest touted alternative therapies. However, scientific studies have never shown that any specific diet alone can control any form of arthritis, with the exception of gout. However, it is undeniably true that your diet affects your *overall* health, and what we eat has been shown to play a role in many disorders. In addition, several research studies indicate that some people with rheumatoid arthritis regularly find that some foods make their symptoms better and others make their symptoms worse. No consistent patterns were identified with all patients.

Ways in which diet might affect your arthritis include the following:

• **Food sensitivities.** A small number of people with arthritis might be sensitive to certain foods that could trigger symptoms or cause them to worsen.
• **Saturated fats.** A diet high in saturated fats or vegetable oils can increase the inflammatory response, thereby contributing to joint and tissue inflammation.
• **Overall health.** Diet affects your overall health, as well as affecting any other diseases or conditions you may have (such as diabetes or heart disease). This, in turn, may affect how your body handles arthritis symptoms.
• **Poor nutrition.** Finally, just having arthritis can make your diet worse. How? You may be unable to shop for and prepare nutritious food for yourself. Pain and fatigue can diminish your appetite, or make it difficult to eat, prepare and chew.

There are many fad diets that claim to alleviate arthritis – everything from fasting to elimination diets (that is, eliminating a certain food or food group from your diet, such as dairy products). The few well-structured research studies concerning diet indicate that what seems to work for one person with rheumatoid arthritis may not work for another. So don't try any extreme dietary changes. If you notice that eating some food makes your arthritis better or worse, don't be afraid to study the situation and act on it.

Your best nutritional bet is to eat the kind of diet recommended by the American Heart Association or the American Cancer Society – one that is low in saturated fats and calories and rich in fruits, vegetables and grains. If you would like to improve or change your diet, consider consulting a registered dietitian. A dietitian can help you change your eating habits, whether your goal is to eat more nutritiously, gain or lose weight, or find out how to prepare easy meals and snacks. The usual fee is about $75 for a one-hour consultation, which may be covered by your insurance. But the real change is up to you – no health professional can control what you eat.

HERBS, SUPPLEMENTS AND "NATURAL" REMEDIES

When it comes to alternative therapies, this category is the largest by far.

Supplements such as herbs, minerals, animal extracts and enzymes – as well as more exotic remedies – are increasingly available to people with chronic health problems such as arthritis. What's more, people are buying and using them in record numbers. In 1998 and 1999, for example, consumers spent approximately $10.4 billion on herbal and dietary supplement products, according to market researchers.

Herbs, supplements and other such "natural" remedies have a tremendous attraction for people with arthritis who are frustrated with the solutions offered by conventional medicine. Although most people realize there is no magic bullet to cure arthritis, they hope their pain and other symptoms will be better controlled if they try a supplement or extract in addition to their formally prescribed medication.

Supplements offer the convenience of popping a pill or potion along with the premise that the natural ingredients won't harm you. But "natural" doesn't always mean "safe." Some people think that supplements – especially herbs – are safe because they are natural alternatives to the chemicals used in prescription drugs. The fact is, herbs *are* chemicals. And anything that's strong enough to help may also be strong enough to hurt.

All this is not to say that supplements are not good. In fact, certain types of extracts and supplements have been shown to be useful in treating various types of arthritis. For example, the omega-3 fatty acids found in the oils from certain fish have been shown to modify inflammation associated with rheumatoid arthritis when taken in large quantities. Unfortunately, the effect may only be sustained for a few months. Another study showed that oil extracted from the borage plant had some properties similar to nonsteroidal anti-inflammatory drugs (NSAIDs), without gastrointestinal side effects. However, the best dosages and possible long-term side effects of these supplements have yet to be determined.

At this point, it is difficult to know the effect of supplements. There is also a phenomenon known as the *placebo effect*. In many research studies, some people are given the actual pill or treatment being tested, while others unknowingly receive a placebo (Latin for "I will please"), an inactive pill or treatment. Some people taking the placebo will experience the same results (reduced pain, for example) as the people taking the real drug, pointing to the potency of the power of suggestion.

For most types of supplements, unfortunately, solid scientific evidence is just not available. Few studies have been done to test supplements, and the studies that do exist usually don't stand up to rigorous scientific examination. In addition, these types of treatments are not regulated and tested in the same way that pharmaceutical products are to ensure that they are both safe and effective. Finally, there are few or no purity standards or quality control mechanisms in place.

It may seem like a paradox, but most pills that are labeled as natural contain chemicals that are processed, just like drugs. It's true that natural substances are chemicals found in the body normally, while drugs are chemicals that are not normally found in the body. But the chemicals in drugs are tested extensively for safety and purity, while the natural pills are not tested on the same level. It's not that you shouldn't consider natural remedies, but you should be aware of the concerns.

If you do decide to try an herbal extract, dietary supplement or other natural remedy, you should proceed with caution and keep the following points in mind:

- **Ask questions.** Don't be afraid to ask your doctor, pharmacist or other health professionals for their opinion or a recommendation.
- **Buy wisely.** When purchasing a supplement, buy from a large company, pharmacy or health-food chain. They may have more stringent quality controls than small companies to maintain their good reputation.
- **Read labels carefully.** Be aware that no supplement can lawfully claim to treat, cure, diagnose or prevent disease. Look for products with the U.S.P. notation, indicating that the manufacturer followed standards established by the United States Pharmacopoeia.
- **Try products one at a time.** If you try only one you can keep track of its effect (or lack of effect). If you notice any side effects, stop taking the supplement right away.

PRAYER AND SPIRITUALITY

Many people believe that prayer and spirituality can help us cope with suffering, offer comfort in times of illness and depression and perhaps even help in healing. Public opinion polls have shown that prayer is one of the most commonly used alternative therapies for arthritis. Indeed, research in behavioral medicine suggests that the interactions of the mind, body and spirit can have powerful effects on our health. But very few published scientific studies have examined the effects of prayer and spirituality.

It may be difficult to measure the effects of prayer and faith on health. One way scientists have approached the issue is to study people who regularly attend religious services, compared with others who do not. Such studies suggest that people who attend religious services tend to live longer, take better care of their health and recover more quickly from illnesses and depression. However, skeptics contend that these studies really show the benefits of companionship and community, not religion.

People have found comfort, meaning and inspiration from prayer and other spiritual practices for thousands of years. Adding or deepening the spiritual aspects in your life could be good for you and arthritis, and – unless you abandon your medication and/or other components of your treatment program – certainly won't hurt you. Just remember that prayer alone will not "cure" your arthritis.

MISCELLANEOUS THERAPIES

Many other types of alternative and complementary therapies are available. In fact, it seems new ones are reported every week. They range from the probably harmless (copper bracelets) to the potentially harmful (bee sting therapy). For a more in-depth look at therapies targeted to people with arthritis, check out *The Arthritis Foundation Guide to Alternative Therapies*, published in 1999.

Learn More About Alternative Therapies

The Arthritis Foundation's Guide to Alternative Therapies ($24.95) offers reliable answers to your questions about nearly 90 different forms of alternative treatments for arthritis, including supplements, acupuncture, tai chi, yoga, chiropractic, meditation, magnet therapy and more. To order the book, call 1-800-207-8633 or visit the Arthritis Foundation's online arthritis store at www.arthritis.org.

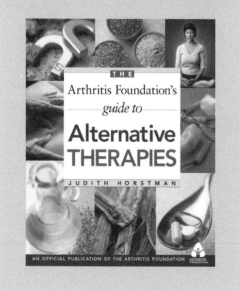

Talking to Your Doctor About Your Options

Doctors are more willing to discuss the use of alternative and complementary therapies with their patients than ever before, in part because they realize that their patients are using them, with or without a doctor's advice. Also, there is strong evidence that many complementary therapies can and do relieve some of the symptoms of arthritis, at least in the short-term.

If your doctor seems reluctant to talk about alternatives to traditional medical treatment with you, don't give up. Tell your doctor that it is important to you to discuss this topic. Be insistent (but not confrontational). The following list of questions might help you open the lines of communication:

- **Is this a therapy that might help my condition?**
- **Have you read any studies about or had experience with this type of therapy?**
- **Is this therapy controversial? Why (or why not)?**
- **What are the hazards of the therapy?**
- **Will there be any interaction between this therapy and the medications or other treatments you have prescribed for me?**
- **Where can I get more information on the therapy?**

Remember, it's in your best interest to keep your doctor informed about your treatment decisions. He or she can't give you the best professional advice without knowing all

Before Trying an Alternative Therapy

- Most alternative therapies are not regulated.

Before you decide to try one of these therapies, find out as much about it as you can. A good source of information is the National Center for Complementary and Alternative Medicine (NCCAM). For a free packet of information on alternative therapies, write to the NCCAM Clearinghouse, P.O. Box 8218, Silver Spring, MD 20807-8218.

- Once you have information on a particular therapy, you may choose to discuss it with your doctor.

He or she will be able to answer important questions such as "How will this affect my treatment plan overall?" and "Could this cause any problems by interacting with my medications?"

- If you decide to proceed, do so with caution.

Seek out a qualified practitioner. For example, there are licensing requirements by state and/or national boards in biofeedback, acupuncture and massage therapy.

- Consider the cost.

Many alternative therapies are expensive, forcing you to weigh your options carefully. Therapies such as massage may or may not be covered by insurance policies when recommended by a physician, so read your policy closely.

- Use good judgment.

If the practitioner makes unrealistic claims (such as, "It will cure your arthritis.") or suggests that you should discontinue your conventional treatment, consider it a strong warning that something is not right.

Adapted from: *Kids Get Arthritis Too.* Atlanta: Arthritis Foundation. May/June 1999.

of the treatments you are using – whether they are over-the-counter drugs, herbal remedies or exercise programs.

Making Smart Choices

Keeping in mind all we've discussed in this chapter, it's up to you to be a smart consumer when it comes to the use of alternative and complementary therapies. Be realistic when assessing the benefits and drawbacks of such therapies. Based on what we know now, certain alternative/complementary practices can help ease some arthritis symptoms, improve your outlook and work with conventional medicine to enhance the effects of your arthritis treatment plan. However, these therapies cannot replace proven medical treatments, nor can they cure chronic disease.

Chapter 18

Good Living:

Creating a Wellness Lifestyle

We have come a long way in this book, and we've covered quite a bit of information — including information to help you understand more about rheumatoid arthritis, the modern treatments available at this time, and practical suggestions that may help make living with rheumatoid arthritis easier. In fact, you may be feeling overwhelmed by the sheer volume of it all, and wondering how you can ever pull it all together into a plan that works for you.

In this chapter, we will try to help you do just that: Take the information that pertains to you and use it to create your own "wellness lifestyle." A wellness lifestyle is one in which you are committed to nourishing your body and mind. It includes attitudes and behaviors that help you achieve the highest possible physical, mental and spiritual well-being. Creating a wellness lifestyle is a cornerstone of being a successful self-manager.

Setting Reasonable Goals

Obviously, there are many components to learning to live well with arthritis, or any other chronic disease. And, as we have stressed throughout this book, no two people are alike and no one experiences rheumatoid arthritis in exactly the same way. Take a few moments to look back over the Table of Contents of this book. Some chapters may not apply to you right now. For example, your active disease may be well controlled by medication, so the chapter on surgery may be of less interest to you at this point. Or perhaps you're into exercise and have already worked out what kinds of exercises make you feel better and which ones to avoid.

Now, jot down a few areas you feel you need to change in your life to achieve a wellness lifestyle. The key word here is "few." How many times have you made sweeping New Year's resolutions, only to break them in a couple of weeks and end up feeling guilty and defeated? Changing old habits and creating new ones is hard work. Most experts advise setting reasonable goals that you can live with, rather than trying to change everything in your life at once. An example of a reasonable goal for yourself might be something like "I will walk three times a week for 20 minutes," rather than "I will begin training to run the New York Marathon!"

You may want to make copies of the form below and use them to draw up weekly contracts with yourself. This will help you set reasonable goals by listing the specific steps you will take to achieve each goal.

Once you accomplish these goals, you can either raise the bar (for example, walking 40 minutes instead of 20), or if you've reached a level that you're happy with, you can turn your attention to other areas.

Nourishing Your Mind and Spirit

When you're setting goals, don't forget about those that will help you keep a healthy mental, as well as physical, outlook. Taking the time to nourish your mind and spirit can lead to unexpected health benefits like less physical pain, something

Contract Form

THIS WEEK I WILL: **WEEK OF:**_____

This week I will walk (what) around the block (how much) before lunch (when) three times (how many).

What

How Much

When

How Many Days

How Certain Are You *(On a scale of 0 to 10 with 0 being totally unsure and 10 being totally confident)*

Signature:

researchers have found repeatedly to be true for people with chronic diseases.

We aren't always taught how to nourish ourselves emotionally or spiritually. Sometimes, people are taught to do the exact opposite – to ignore their emotions or feelings. But there are many ways that we can enrich our minds and spirits. Consider the following points to support a healthy mental outlook.

- **Optimism.** Having the view that things in general are pretty good can help you live longer and reduce chronic stress. Expect good things to happen, and work toward them. Stop worrying so much! Live one day at a time and use relaxation techniques and healthy self-talk to counter pessimistic thoughts.

- **Humor.** Laughter really is good medicine. Author Norman Cousins refers to laughing as "internal jogging." Anything that makes you smile brings relief to your mind and spirit. Some research has shown that humor may even improve your immune function.

- **Sense of purpose.** Do you believe you have worth and that there is a purpose for your life and experiences? People who believe in themselves and in the meaning of their lives are happier, more satisfied and

Personally Speaking Stories from real people with rheumatoid arthritis

"I wake up to a beautiful spring day. The sun is shining, a warm breeze is blowing, squirrels are playing tag. A rabbit nibbles clover while the blue jay in the pine tree outside my window scolds him. All these things, in addition to walking, I used to take for granted.

Smelling the Roses, Watching the Clouds – Appreciating Life
by Suzie Hershman, Matawan, NJ

"A few years ago, I had 'routine' hip replacement surgery and almost ended up being unable to walk. Several surgeries and thousands of hours of physical therapy later, I'm walking! The time span and length of my walks are still limited; I will never be as strong or as stable was I was before. This can be depressing. When I lose patience and feel like giving up, I talk to a friend who reminds me how far I've come, and how much better I'm doing. Often, I write lists of things I can or cannot do. I compare the recent lists with the old lists. Looking at the improvements I've made, written down on paper, makes them seem more tangible.

"I stop and smell the roses that my husband planted along our driveway. I admire the splendid pinks, reds and oranges in the setting sun. I look out my window while typing, and watch the billowy, white clouds float across the sky. There are many other wonderful things in my world that help me get through the tough days, as well as the good ones."

serene. This belief in one's self is a choice that occurs regardless of life circumstances.

• **Sense of control.** Do you feel hopeless or frustrated by your arthritis or by other challenges in your life? Given the same situation, some people will feel helpless, and others feel a sense of control or of confidence that they can influence their own well-being. Goal setting, problem solving, self-monitoring, and communicating your needs and feelings to others are all ways to help you regain a sense of control.

• **Social support.** Is your life filled with satisfying relationships and love? Do you feel that others understand your arthritis and the demands it places on you? Getting the support you need can be hard work. You need to be a friend to have a friend. You need to be willing to listen to others and communicate your own needs in a clear, direct way.

Taking Care of the Basics

To truly live well with rheumatoid arthritis, you should take steps toward healthy living in general. Most of these basics have already been discussed in this book, but they're worth repeating because they are such an important part of feeling healthy and in charge of your life. So keep them in mind as you build your wellness lifestyle:

• **Eat a healthy diet.** Most people with rheumatoid arthritis don't need to follow any special diet. However, you should try to follow the guidelines for a healthy diet described on page 183, or explained in the USDA's food pyramid found on many packaged foods, like dry cereals.

• **Get enough sleep.** Many people are sleep-deprived due to the demands of work, family and other obligations. We rise early and don't get to bed until late. Lack of sleep increases stress levels and may decrease your body's immune activity. Review the suggestions in Chapter 16 for getting a good night's sleep.

• **Manage stress in healthy ways.** We've talked about ways to reduce stress levels and tips for handling those stresses that can't be eliminated (see Chapter 13). Resist the temptation to handle stress in unhealthy ways – such as overeating, over-indulging in alcohol or taking drugs – that will only increase stress in the long run.

• **Balance exercise and rest.** Getting regular exercise should be an important part of your wellness lifestyle, but don't forget to balance periods of activity with periods of rest. Taking a 20-minute breather may feel like a waste of time, but it may just give you the energy you need to make it through the day.

A Final Word: Making Time for Yourself

Too many people fall into the trap of doing everything that others expect of them but failing to leave enough time for themselves. However, research has shown that your use of time and your overall balance of activities can affect your health and satisfaction with life. Try using the Time Target at the end of this chapter to help you think about how satisfied you are with the amount

Guidelines for a Healthy Diet

Eat a variety of foods.

Maintain a healthy weight.

Cut down on fat and cholesterol consumption.

Eat plenty of vegetables, fruits and grain products.

Use sugar and salt in moderation.

Drink plenty of water – most experts recommend eight glasses per day.

If you drink alcohol, do so in moderation.

of time you now spend on activities such as hobbies, time alone or with friends, or other activities that are just for you.

Look for patterns in the Time Target. Is your life balanced so that most or all of the "bull's eye" (the center circle) is colored in? Or do you have a lot of parts of the other circles colored in? Look for colored areas in these outer circles:

• **"Need Less" circle.** If you have a lot of this circle colored in, you may have trouble setting priorities or saying no to others. Are you feeling overwhelmed? If so, go back and read the strategies for dealing with fatigue in Chapter 16, and for using more effective self-management techniques in Chapter 13.

• **"Need More" circle.** Is it hard for you to ask for what you need? Do you need more from people in relationships? You may need to practice better planning so that you can spend more time on more enjoyable activities.

Remember to set goals, contract, problem solve and plan to get where you want to be.

• **"Not Important" circle.** If you have colored five or more of the activities as "not important," this may be a sign that you are feeling depressed. If you've lost interest in many activities that you used to enjoy, if you've isolated yourself from friends, or if you feel like hurting yourself, seek professional help. Go back and review the sections on coping with stress and coping with depression in Chapter 13 for additional help.

It is important to find those things in life that uplift and bring joy and happiness to your life. This will take time, patience and determination, but if you can learn to balance each of the hassles in your life with uplifting activities, rheumatoid arthritis can become just a part of your life, not your whole life.

Remember: Aim for the bull's eye.

Targeting Your Time

Instructions: Read the names for each of the 12 activities listed in the wedges of the circle below. Think about how satisfied you are with the time you now spend on each activity. Color in the part of the wedge for each activity that best describes how that activity fits into your life. For example, if you are satisfied with time spent on an activity, color the center part of the wedge, in the "OK" section. Otherwise, indicate by coloring whether you "need less" or "need more" of the activity, or if the activity is "not important" in your life.

HOW CLOSE ARE YOU TO THE BULL'S-EYE?

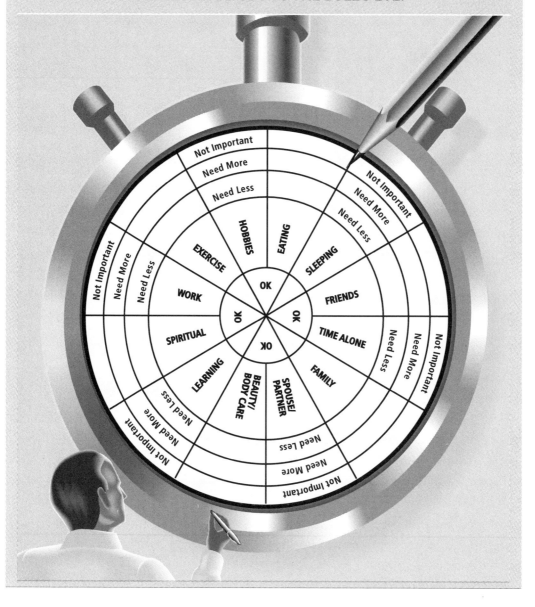

GLOSSARY

acupressure: Eastern medicine technique in which pressure is applied to specific sites along energy pathways called meridians.

acupuncture: Eastern medicine technique in which needles are used to puncture the body at specific sites along energy pathways called meridians.

acute illness: Disease that can be severe, but is of short duration, unlike chronic illness.

acute pain: See *pain*.

adrenal glands: Glands located near the kidneys. These glands secrete a variety of hormones, including glucocorticoids.

adrenaline: A hormone that increases the heart and respiration rate when we feel frightened, threatened or angry, preparing us to flee to safety, or stand and fight.

aerobic: An activity designed to increase oxygen consumption by the body, such as aerobic exercise or aerobic breathing.

alternative therapy: Any practice or substance outside the realm of conventional medicine.

American College of Rheumatology (ACR): An organization that provides a professional, educational and research forum for rheumatologists across the country. Among its functions is helping determine what symptoms and signs define the various types of rheumatic disease diagnoses and what the appropriate treatments are for those diagnoses.

analgesic: Drugs used to help relieve pain.

anemia: A condition marked by a reduction in the number of red blood cells, amount of hemoglobin in the blood, or total blood volume.

anemia, iron deficiency: Anemia resulting from a greater demand on the stored iron than can be supplied.

anemia, pernicious: Anemia resulting from a lack of vitamin B-12; it is associated with absence of hydrochloric acid in the stomach.

anesthesia: Chemicals that induce a partial or complete loss of sensation. Used to perform surgery and other medical procedures.

anesthesiologist: A physician specializing in the administration of anesthesia.

ankylosing spondylitis: Form of arthritis that primarily affects the joints and ligaments of the spine, marked by pain and stiffness. Can result in fusion of joints and bones, leading to rigidity.

antibody: A specialized protein that neutralizes *antigens*, or foreign substances, in the body.

antigen: A foreign substance that begins an immune reaction in the body.

antinuclear antibody test: Test used to detect presence of abnormal antibodies.

arthritis: From the Greek word "arth" meaning "joint," and the suffix "itis" meaning "inflammation." It generally means involvement of a joint from any cause, such as infection, trauma or inflammation.

arthrodesis: A surgical procedure involving the fusing of two bones.

arthroplasty: A surgical procedure to replace a joint with an artificial one.

arthroscopic surgery: A type of surgery using

an instrument, called an arthroscope, consisting of a thin tube with a light at one end, inserted into the body through a small incision, and connected to a closed-circuit television.

aspiration: The removal of a substance by suction. Technique used to remove fluid from an inflamed joint, both to relieve pressure and to examine the fluid.

autoantibody: antibodies acting against the body's own tissues.

autoimmune disorder: An illness in which the body's immune system mistakenly attacks and damages tissues of the body. There are many types of autoimmune disorders, including arthritis and the rheumatic diseases.

biologic response modifiers: Drugs that target the specific components of the immune system that contribute to disease. Includes etanercept and infliximab.

biomedical model: Traditional model of medical care, based on the principle of identifying a single cause and cure for each disease.

biopsychosocial model: More recent model of medical care, where patient's self-management plays a part in treatment of chronic disease, and where biological, psychological and socioeconomic factors are considered influential to the disease's outcome.

body mechanics: The structures and methods with which your body moves and performs physical tasks.

bone densitometry: Imaging study used to measure bone density, particularly in diagnosing osteoporosis.

bunion: Inflammation, enlargement and malalignment of the joint of the great toe.

bursa: A small sac located between a tendon and a bone. The bursae (plural for bursa) reduce friction and provide lubrication. See also *bursitis*.

bursitis: Inflammation of a bursa (see above), which can occur when the joint has been overused or when the joint has become deformed by arthritis. Bursitis makes it painful to move or put pressure on the affected joint.

C-reactive protein: Protein that when found in elevated levels in the body is an indication of inflammation.

capsaicin: A chemical contained in some hot peppers. Capsaicin gives these peppers their "burn" and has painkilling properties. It is available in nonprescription creams that can be rubbed on the skin over a joint to relieve pain.

cartilage: A firm, smooth, rubbery substance that provides a gliding surface for joint motion, and prevents bone-on-bone contact.

chiropodist: a doctor with particular training in the care of the feet. Also called *podiatrist*.

chronic illness: Disease that is of a long duration, such as rheumatoid arthritis.

chronic pain: Pain that is constant or persists over a long period of time, perhaps throughout life. See *pain*.

circadian rhythm: The daily, monthly and seasonal schedules on which living things carry out essential biologic tasks, such as eating, digesting, eliminating, growing and resting. Disruption of these rhythms

– when you travel rapidly across time zones (promoting "jet lag"), for example – has a negative and sometimes profound impact on performance and mood.

complementary therapy: Any practice or substance used in conjunction with traditional treatment.

control group: A group of people used as a standard for comparison in scientific studies.

cool-down exercises: A series of physical activities that allow your heart and respiration rates to return to normal after being elevated by exercise.

corticosteroids: See *glucocorticoids*.

cortisone: A hormone produced by the cortex of the adrenal gland. Cortisone has potent anti-inflammatory effects but can also have side effects. See also *glucocorticoids*.

Cox-2 inhibitors: Drugs that inhibit inflammation without the gastrointestinal side effects of traditional NSAIDs. Includes celecoxib and rofecoxib.

cytokines: Chemicals involved in the inflammatory response.

cytotoxic drugs: Chemicals that destroy cells or prevent their multiplication.

deconditioning: Loss of muscle mass and strength because of inactivity. See also *reconditioning*.

deep breathing: Drawing air into the lungs, filling them as much as possible, and then exhaling slowly. Performing this type of breathing rhythmically for a few minutes increases the amount of oxygen refreshing your brain and produces relaxation and readiness for mental tasks.

depression: A state of mind characterized by gloominess, dejection or sadness.

depression, clinical: A recognized mental illness in which the feelings of depression are severe, prolonged and hamper your ability to function normally.

dermatomyositis: See *polymyositis*.

disease: Sickness. Some physicians use this term only for conditions in which a structural or functional change in tissues or organs has been identified.

disorder: An ailment; an abnormal health condition.

DMARDs: Disease modifying antirheumatic drugs, used to slow or stop the progression of inflammatory joint disease. Includes methotrexate.

dose-pack: A package of glucocorticoid drugs with a tapered daily dosage.

double-blind studies: A method used in scientific studies to compare one intervention (such as a new medication) with other interventions, or no intervention. In this method, the study participants and the persons evaluating the interventions are "blinded" – that is, they aren't told who is getting the intervention being tested – so their responses will not be influenced by their opinions or expectations of the intervention.

endorphins: Natural painkillers produced by the human nervous system that have qualities similar to opiate drugs. Endorphins are released during exercise and when we laugh.

endurance exercises: Exercises such as swimming,

walking and cycling that use the large muscles of the body and are dependent on increasing the amount of oxygen that reaches the muscles. These exercises strengthen muscles and increase and maintain physical fitness.

enthesis: The place where the tendon inserts into the bone.

ergonomics: The study of human capabilities and limitations in relation to the work system, machine or task, as well as the study of the physical, psychological and social environment of the worker. Also known as "human engineering."

erosions: Small holes near the ends of bones.

erythrocyte sedimentation rate: A test measuring how fast red blood cells (erythrocytes) fall to the bottom of a test tube, indicating level of inflammation. Often called ESR or "sed rate."

fatigue: A general worn-down feeling of no energy. Fatigue can be caused by excessive physical, mental or emotional exertion, by lack of sleep, and by inflammation or disease.

Felty's syndrome: Form of rheumatoid arthritis marked by an enlargement of the spleen and a reduced number of white blood cells.

fibromyalgia: A noninfectious rheumatic condition affecting the body's soft tissue. Characterized by muscle pain, fatigue and nonrestorative sleep, fibromyalgia produces no abnormal X-ray or laboratory findings. It is often associated with headaches and irritable bowel syndrome.

flare: A term used to describe times when the disease or condition is at its worst.

flexibility exercises: Muscle stretches and other activities designed to maintain flexibility and to prevent stiffness or shortening of ligaments and tendons.

Food Labeling Act: Recent legal decree of the U.S. government mandating the type of information that must be given on food labels regarding nutritional content. This act ensures that consumers will have easy-to-read fat, protein, fiber, carbohydrate and calorie content information, and more.

gate theory: A theory of how pain signals travel to the brain. According to this theory, pain signals must pass a "pain gate" that can be opened or closed by various positive (e.g., feelings of happiness) or negative (e.g., feelings of sadness) factors.

genetic predisposition: Susceptibility to a specific disease or illness caused by certain inherited characteristics.

glucocorticoids: A group of hormones including cortisol produced by the adrenal glands. They can also be synthetically produced (that is, made in a laboratory) and have powerful anti-inflammatory effects. These drugs are sometimes called corticosteroids or steroids, but they are not the same as the dangerous performance-enhancing drugs that some athletes use to promote strength and endurance.

gout: Disease that occurs due to an excess of uric acid in the blood, causing crystals to deposit in the joint, leading to pain and inflammation.

grief: Feelings of loss; acute sorrow.

guided imagery: A method of managing pain and stress. Following the voice of a "guide," an audiotape or videotape, or one's own internal voice, attention is focused on a series of images that lead one's mind away from the stressor or pain.

H2 blockers: Compounds that act by blocking receptors in the stomach that lead to the production of acid.

hammer toes: A specific type of joint malalignment of the toes seen in rheumatoid arthritis.

helplessness: The concept of not feeling in control of your life or your health.

hematocrit: The percentage of red blood cells found in blood.

hemoglobin: The protein in red blood cells that carries oxygen from the lungs to the tissues.

hormones: Concentrated chemical substances produced in the glands or organs that have specific – and usually multiple – regulatory effects to carry out in the body.

illness: Poor health; sickness.

immune response: Activation of the body's immune system.

immune system: Your body's complex biochemical system for defending itself against bacteria, viruses, wounds and other injuries. Among the many components of the system are a variety of cells (such as T cells), organs (such as the lymph glands) and chemicals (such as histamine and prostaglandins).

inflammation: A response to injury or infection that involves a sequence of biochemical reactions. Inflammation can be generalized, causing fatigue, fever, and pain or tenderness all over the body. It can also be localized, for example, in joints, where it causes swelling and pain. In rheumatoid arthritis, inflammation is not caused by injury or infection, but is part of an autoimmune reaction.

internist: A physician who specializes in internal medicine; sometimes called a primary-care physician.

isometric exercises: Exercises that build the muscles around joints by tightening the muscles without moving the joints.

isotonic exercises: Exercises that strengthen muscles by moving the joints.

joint: The place or part where one bone connects to another.

joint count: An examination done by a doctor to determine the number of joints that are affected by arthritis.

joint malalignment: When joints are not aligned properly, due to joint damage.

joint replacement surgery: Also known as *arthroplasty*, a surgical procedure involving the reconstruction or replacement (with a man-made component) of a joint.

ligament: Flexible band of fibrous tissue that connects bones to one another.

locus: The site of a gene on a chromosome.

lupus (systemic lupus erythematosus): The term used to describe an inflammatory connective tissue autoimmune disease that can involve the skin, joints, kidneys, blood and other organs, and is associated with antinuclear antibodies.

malalignment, joint: When joints are not aligned properly, due to joint damage.

massage: A technique of applying pressure, friction or vibration to the muscles, by hand or using a massage appliance, to stimulate circulation and produce relaxation and pain relief.

massage therapist: One who has completed a program of study and is licensed to perform massage.

meditation: A sustained period of deep inward thought, reflection and openness to inspiration.

meridians: Energy pathways used in Eastern medicine, but that have no Western medicine counterparts.

morbidity (rate): The frequency or proportion of people with a particular diagnosis or disability in a given population.

MRI: Magnetic Resonance Imaging test, a scan used as a diagnostic aid.

muscle: Tissue that moves organs or parts of the body.

myalgia: Pain of the muscles.

narcotics: A class of drugs that reduce pain by blocking signals traveling from the central nervous system to the brain. While narcotics have the potential to be addictive and are abused by some people, they can be used safely for effective pain relief under skilled medical supervision.

NSAID (nonsteroidal anti-inflammatory drug): A type of drug that does not contain steroids but is used to relieve pain and reduce inflammation.

nurse: A person who has received education and training in health care, particularly patient care.

nurse practitioner: A registered nurse with advanced training and emphasis in primary care.

objective: Capable of being observed or measured; for example, infection can be objectively observed by the presence of bacteria in a blood test or culture test. See also *subjective*.

occupational therapist: A health professional who teaches patients to reduce strain on joints while doing everyday activities.

orthopaedic surgeon: A surgeon who specializes in diseases of the bone.

orthopaedist: A physician who specializes in diseases of the bone.

osteoarthritis: A disease causing cartilage breakdown in certain joints (spine, hands, hips, knees) resulting in pain and deformity.

osteoporosis: A disease that causes bones to lose their mass and break easily.

osteotomy: A surgical procedure involving the cutting of bone, usually performed in cases of severe joint malalignment.

pain: A sensation or perception of hurting, ranging from discomfort to agony, that occurs in response to injury, disease or functional disorder. Pain is your body's alarm system, signaling that something is wrong. *Acute* pain is temporary and related to nerve endings stimulated by tissue damage and improves with healing. *Chronic* pain may be mild to severe but persists due to prolonged tissue damage or due to pain impulses that keep the pain gate open.

palindromic rheumatism: Self-limited attacks of joint inflammation that occur every few weeks or months, then subside after a few days. About one half of people who experience palindromic rheumatism go on to develop chronic rheumatoid arthritis.

pediatrician: A physician with special training who specializes in the diagnosis, treatment and prevention of childhood and adolescent illness.

pediatric rheumatologist: See *rheumatologist*.

peptic ulcer: A benign (not cancerous) lesion in the stomach or duodenum that may cause pain, nausea, vomiting or bleeding. Such lesions can be caused by nonsteroidal anti-inflammatory drugs such as aspirin or ibuprofen.

pericarditis: Inflammation of the lining surrounding the heart.

pharmacist: A professional licensed to prepare and dispense drugs.

physiatrist: A physician who continues training after medical school and specializes in the field of physical medicine and rehabilitation.

physical therapist: A person who has professional training and is licensed in the practice of physical therapy.

physical therapy: Methods and techniques of rehabilitation to restore function and prevent disability following injury or disease. Methods may include applications of heat and cold, assistive devices, massage, and an individually tailored program of exercises.

physician: A person who has successfully completed medical school and is licensed to practice medicine.

physician, family: See *physician, primary care*.

physician, general practitioner: See *physician, primary care*.

physician, primary care: Physician to whom a family or individual goes initially when ill or for a periodic health check. This physician assumes medical coordination of care with other physicians for the patient with multiple health concerns.

physician's assistant: A person trained, certified and licensed to assist physicians by recording medical history and performing the physical examination, diagnosis and treatment of commonly encountered medical problems under the supervision of a licensed physician.

placebo effect: The phenomenon in which a person receiving an inactive drug or therapy experiences a reduction in symptoms.

platelets: Small cells that participate in the formation of blood clotting.

pleurisy: Inflammation of the lining of the lungs.

podagra: Gout occurring in the big toe.

podiatrist: A health professional who specializes in care of the foot. Formerly called a *chiropodist*.

polyarthritis: Arthritis affecting many joints.

polymyositis: Disease in which inflammation occurs primarily in the muscles, leading to muscle weakness and permanent muscle damage. Often associated with dermatomyositis, a condition marked by skin rashes.

Prosorba column: Treatment in which certain

antibodies associated with rheumatoid arthritis are removed from the blood using a special filtering machine.

proton pump inhibitors: Drugs that block the secretion of acid into the stomach, used to protect the stomach against the gastrointestinal side effects associated with NSAIDs.

psoriatic arthritis: A condition in which psoriasis (a common skin disease) occurs in conjunction with the inflammation of arthritis.

psychiatrist: A physician who trains after medical school in the study, treatment and prevention of mental disorders. A psychiatrist may provide counseling and prescribe medicines and other therapies.

psychologist: A trained professional, usually a PhD rather than an MD, who specializes in the mind and mental processes, especially in relation to human and animal behavior. A psychologist may measure mental abilities and provide counseling.

psychosomatic: Pertaining to the link between the mind (psyche) and the body (soma).

pulmonary fibrosis: Scarring of the lungs, leading to shortness of breath.

radiograph: An X-ray.

range of motion: The distance and angles at which your joints can be moved, extended and rotated in various directions.

Raynaud's phenomenon: Restriction of blood flow to the fingers, toes, or (rarely) to the nose or ears, in response to cold or emotional upset. This results in temporary blanching or paleness of the skin, tingling, numbness and pain.

reconditioning: Restoring or improving muscle tone and strength with appropriate and balanced exercise, nutrition and rest. See also *deconditioning*.

rehabilitation counselor: A person who guides physical and mental rehabilitation.

relaxation: A state of release from mental or physical stress or tension.

remission: The term used to describe a period when symptoms of a disease or condition improve or even disappear.

remodeling: The regrowth of bone around an artificial joint.

resection: Surgical procedure involving removing all or part of a bone.

resection arthroplasty: A surgical procedure in which resection is done in conjunction with arthroplasty.

revision: A surgical procedure to replace an artificial joint.

rheumatic disease: A general term referring to conditions characterized by pain and stiffness of the joints or muscles. The American College of Rheumatology currently recognizes over 100 rheumatic diseases. The term is often used interchangeably with "arthritis" (meaning joint inflammation), but not all rheumatic diseases affect the joints or involve inflammation.

rheumatoid arthritis: A chronic, inflammatory autoimmune disease in which the body's protective immune system turns on the body and attacks the joints, causing pain, swelling and deformity.

rheumatoid factor: An abnormal antibody often found in blood of people with rheumatoid arthritis.

rheumatoid nodules: Lumps of tissue that form under the skin, often over bony areas exposed to pressure, such as on the fingers or around the elbow.

rheumatologist: A physician who pursues additional training after medical school and specializes in the diagnosis, treatment and prevention of arthritis and other rheumatic disorders.

rheumatologist, pediatric: A rheumatologist who specializes in the diagnosis, treatment and prevention of arthritis or other rheumatic diseases in children and adolescents.

salicylates: A subcategory of NSAIDs, including aspirin.

scleritis: Inflammation of the eyes.

scleroderma: A connective tissue disease characterized by a tightening of the skin, and a discoloration of the hands when exposed to cold (known as Raynaud's phenomenon). Can affect internal organs as well.

scleromalacia perforans: Permanent eye damage caused by severe inflammation.

self-efficacy: The concept of a person having emotional control in reaction to events in their life, such as a chronic illness.

self-help: Any course, activity, or action that you do for yourself to improve your circumstances or ability to cope with a situation.

self-management: The concept of a person having control of his or her disease and its management.

self-talk: The voice in your head that you use to talk to yourself, out loud or in thought.

shared epitope: Genetic marker that approximately two-thirds of people with rheuma-

toid arthritis have.

Sjögren's syndrome: Syndrome affecting the salivary and lacrimal (tear-producing) glands, leading to dry eyes and dry mouth.

skeletal muscles: The voluntary muscles that are primarily involved in moving parts of the body. "Voluntary" in this sense refers to muscles that move in response to our decisions to walk, bend, grasp and so on, as opposed to muscles such as the heart, which do their work without our willful direction.

social worker: A person who has professional training and is licensed to assist people in need by helping them capitalize on their own resources and connecting them with social services (for example, home nursing care or vocational rehabilitation).

soft-tissue rheumatism: Pertaining to the many rheumatic conditions affecting the soft (as opposed to the hard or bony) tissues of the body. Fibromyalgia is one type of soft-tissue rheumatism. Others are bursitis, tendinitis and focal myofascial pain.

spontaneous remission: A somewhat rare disappearance of symptoms of rheumatoid arthritis, usually occurring in the early stage of disease.

steroids: A group name for lipids (fat substances) produced in the body and sharing a particular type of chemical structure. Among these are bile acids, cholesterol and some hormones. Not the same as anabolic steroids, drugs synthesized from testosterone (the male sex hormone), and used by some athletes to promote strength and endurance.

strain: Injury to a muscle, tendon or ligament

by repetitive use, trauma or excessive stretching.

strengthening exercises: Exercises that help maintain or increase muscle strength. See also *isometric exercises* and *isotonic exercises*.

stress: The body's physical, mental and chemical reactions to frightening, exciting, dangerous or irritating circumstances.

stressor: Factors that cause stress in your life.

symmetric arthritis: Arthritis affecting the same joints on both sides of the body.

syndrome: A collection of symptoms and/or physical findings that characterize a particular abnormal condition or illness.

synovectomy: Surgical removal of the synovium, or the lining of the joint.

synovitis: Inflammation of the lining of the joint.

synovium: The lining of the joint.

synovial fluid: The fluid found in the joint.

systemic disease: A disease that may affect more than one system in the body.

target heart rate: The number of heartbeats per minute that people want to reach during exercise in order to gain maximum benefits. Because the normal heart rate changes as we age, target heart rates are grouped by age.

tendinitis: Inflammation of a tendon.

tendon: A cord of dense, fibrous tissue uniting a muscle to a bone.

TENS: a treatment for pain involving a small device that directs mild electric pulses to nerves in the painful area.

teratogenic: Causing the malformation of a fetus.

thrombocytopenia: Decreased number of platelets.

tissue: A collection of similar cells that act together to perform a specific function in the body. The primary tissues are epithelial (skin), connective (ligaments and tendons), bone, muscle and nervous.

titer: A standard of strength per volume or units per volume.

trochanteric bursitis: Irritation of the trochanteric bursa, which is located on the bony prominence of the femur or thigh. See also *bursitis*.

Type I disease: Term used in rheumatoid arthritis to describe a case where a person meets certain criteria or shows symptoms of the disease for a short period of time, but these symptoms do not last long or progress in severity.

Type II disease: Term used in rheumatoid arthritis to describe a case where a person meets the criteria for the disease, experiences inflammation in symmetrical joints for longer than six months, and does not experience spontaneous remission of symptoms. A mild disease course that can be controlled with less aggressive therapy.

Type III disease: Most severe form of rheumatoid arthritis, with greater severity of symptoms than Type II disease, requiring aggressive therapy.

uric acid: Substance formed when the body breaks down waste products called purines. Uric acid crystals deposited in the joints cause gout.

urinalysis: Test done on the urine to detect

levels of sugar, protein or abnormal cells.

vasculitis: Inflammation of the blood vessels.

visual analogue scale: A tool used to measure subjective feelings such as pain on a scale of 0 to 10 or 0 to 100.

visualization: A method of thinking that engages the imagination to help you achieve a goal.

warm-up: Gentle movement to warm up the muscles before performing stretches and more strenuous exercise.

INDEX

INDEX

INDEX

INDEX

INDEX

INDEX

RESOURCES

The Arthritis Foundation, the only national, voluntary health organization that works for the more than 43 million Americans with arthritis or related diseases, offers many valuable resources through more than 150 offices nationwide. The chapter that serves your area has information, products, classes and other services to help you take control of your arthritis.

To find the office near you, call 800/283-7800 or search the Arthritis Foundation Web site at www.arthritis.org.

Programs and Services

1. Physician referral – Most Arthritis Foundation chapters can provide a list of local doctors who specialize in the evaluation and treatment of arthritis and arthritis-related diseases.

2. Exercise programs – The Arthritis Foundation sponsors, develops and coordinates exercise programs for people with arthritis, featuring specially-trained instructors.

They include:

• *Joint Efforts:* These classes feature undemanding exercises for all people with arthritis, including those in wheelchairs or walkers.

• *PACE®* (People With Arthritis Can Exercise): These courses feature gentle movements to increase joint flexibility, range of motion, stamina and muscle strength. An accompanying video is available for home use.

• *Arthritis Foundation Aquatics Program:* These water exercise programs help relieve strain on muscles and joints. An accompanying PEP (Pool Exercise Program) video is available for home use.

3. Educational and Support Groups – The Arthritis Foundation sponsors mutual-support groups that provide opportunities for discussion and problem-solving among people with arthritis. In addition, the Arthritis Foundation offers three courses designed to help people actively manage their particular disease through exercise, medications, relaxation techniques, pain management, nutrition and more:

• Arthritis Self-Help Course

• Fibromyalgia Self-Help Course

• Systemic Lupus Erythematosus Self-Help Course

Information and Products

Find the latest information about arthritis, including research, medications, government advocacy, programs and services through the Arthritis Foundation's many information resources.

1. www.arthritis.org -- Information about arthritis is available 24 hours a day on the Internet at the Arthritis Foundation's interactive, comprehensive Web site. Find news about arthritis, ways to get involved, and the Arthritis Store.

2. Arthritis Answers – Call toll-free at 800/283-7800 for 24-hour, automated information about arthritis and Arthritis Foundation resources. Trained volunteers and staff are also available at your local Arthritis Foundation chapter to answer questions or refer you to physicians and other resources. For general information about arthritis, call 404/872-7100 ext. 1, or email questions to help@arthritis.org.

3. Publications – The Arthritis Foundation offers many publications about diagnosis, medications, exercise, diet, pain management and more for people with arthritis.

• *Books* – The Arthritis Foundation publishes a variety of books on arthritis to help you learn to understand and manage your condition, live a healthier life, and cope with the emotional challenges that come with a chronic illness. Order books directly at www.arthritis.org or by calling 800/207-8633. All Arthritis Foundation books are available at many bookstores.

• *Brochures* – The Arthritis Foundation offers brochures containing concise, understandable information on many arthritis topics, including surgery, the latest medications, working with your doctors and self-managing your illness. Single copies are available free of charge at www.arthritis.org or by calling 800/283-7800.

• *Arthritis Today* – This award-winning bimonthly magazine provides the latest information on research, new treatments, trends and tips from experts and readers to help you manage arthritis. A one-year subscription to *Arthritis Today* is included when you become a member of the Arthritis Foundation. Annual membership is $20 and helps fund research to find cures for arthritis. Call 800/933-0032 for information.

• *Newsletters* – Subscribe to the award-winning, up-to-date newsletters *Kids Get Arthritis, Too* (for juvenile arthritis) by calling 800/268-6942, or the *Fibromyalgia Health Letter* by calling 877/775-0343.

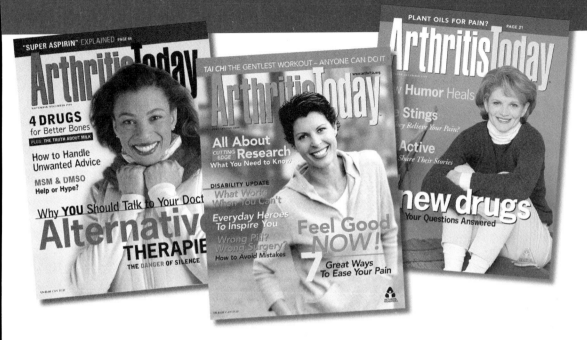
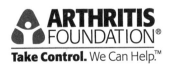

DON'T MISS THESE OTHER GREAT RESOURCES!

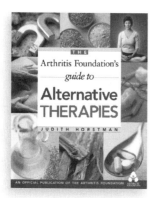

The Arthritis Foundation's Guide to Alternative Therapies

Learn the scientific facts behind the claims about alternative therapies for arthritis, from glucosamine to acupuncture to bee sting therapy and more. Find the therapies that really work.

285 pages
#835-220
$24.95

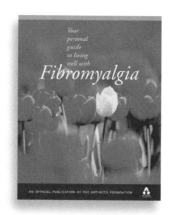

Your Personal Guide to Living Well with Fibromyalgia

This hands-on work-book gives you the tools you need to take control over your condition and start down the path toward wellness.

224 pages
#835-203
$14.95

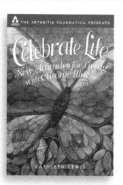

Celebrate Life: New Attitudes for Living with Chronic Illness

Remake your life after diagnosis with help from a health professional who lives with chronic illness herself.

240 pages
#835-219
$12.95

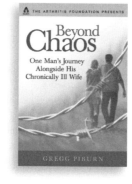

Beyond Chaos: One Man's Journey Alongside His Chronically Ill Wife

Discover how one man turned his frustration and anger about chronic illness into an opportunity to bring a new level of trust and intimacy to his marriage.

346 pages
#835-214
$14.95

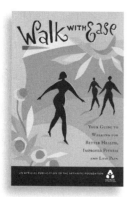

Walk With Ease: Your Guide to Walking For Better Health, Improved Fitness and Less Pain

Create your personal walking program with help from the Stanford Center for Research in Disease Prevention – a great guide to boosting energy, reducing stress and controlling weight.

104 pages
#835-216
$8.95

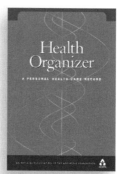

Health Organizer: A Personal Health-Care Record

Track your symptoms and your disease activity in this spiral-bound, tabbed personal journal. Includes a place to keep medical records, daily reminders, a glossary of key terms and important resources.

144 pages
#835-207
$11.95

DON'T WAIT—ORDER TODAY!

1-800-207-8633 (Monday-Friday, 8 a.m.-6p.m. EST)
or www. arthritis.org

Source Code:OABPAGE

ARTHRIT
FOUNDATIC
Take Control. We Can H